RAGING TWENTIES

PEPE ESCOBAR

NIMBLE BOOKS LLC

Copyright © 2021 Pepe Escobar
All rights reserved.
ISBN: 9781608882205

DEDICATION

To Ayan, born 2015

Table of Contents

1. Introduction 1
2. It's The Us Vs. Russia-China-Iran 5
3. The siren call of a "system leader" 11
4. The Westlessness myth 17
5. We are all Stoics now 21
6. Who profits from this controlled demolition? 27
7. Ground control to Planet Lockdown: this is only a test 35
8. How The Riddler may teach us to fight a disease 45
9. Total system failure or the birth of a new economy? 49
10. How Confucius, Buddha and the Tao are winning this "war" 53
11. The City in a Time of Plague 57
12. How to think post-Planet Lockdown 63
13. The deeper roots of Chinese demonization 73
14. The lessons Xi learned from the Ming dynasty 79
15. How biosecurity is enabling digital neo-feudalism 87
16. Our grim future: Restored Neoliberalism or Hybrid Neofascism? 93
17. Barbarism begins at home 99
18. Eurasia, The Hegemon, and The Three Sovereigns 105

19. Clash of civilizations, revisited 121
20. Shadowplay revisited: how Eurasia is being reshaped...... 127
21. From 9/11 to The Great Reset 133
22. The Russia-China vote... 141
23. Flying Dragon, Crashing Eagle... 145
24. Our Techno-Feudal World 149
25. Kim No-VAX Does DARPA.. 155
26. Soleimani geopolitics, one year on..................................... 161

RAGING TWENTIES

Table of Abbreviations

ADB	Asian Development Bank
AI	Artificial Intelligence
AIIB	Asia Infrastructure Investment Bank
AKP	Adalet ve Kalkınma Partisi)
APEC	Asia-Pacific Economic Cooperation
ASEAN	Association of Southeast Asian Nations
BHL	Bernard-Henri Lévy
BRI	Belt and Road Initiative
BRICS	Brazil, Russia, India, China, and South
CCP	Chinese Communist Party
CDC	Centers for Disease Control
CEPI	Coalition for Epidemic Preparedness Innovations
CIPS	Cross-Border Inter-Bank Payments System
CNRS	Centre national de la recherche scientifique
CPEC	China-Pakistan Economic Corridor
CPTPP	Comprehensive and Progressive Agreement for Trans-Pacific Partnership
DARPA	Defense Advanced Research Projects Agency
ECB	European Central Bank
EAEU	Eurasia Economic Union
FOIA	Freedom of Information Act
GDP	Gross domestic product
GWOT	Global War on Terror
GWOV	Global War on Virus
ILO	International Labour Organization
IMF	International Monetary Fund
INSTC	International North South Transportation

		Corridor
	IoT	Internet of things
	IRGC	Islamic Revolutionary Guards Corps
	ISIS	Islamic State of Iraq and Syria
	JCPOA	Joint Comprehensive Plan of Action
	MAD	Mutually assured destruction
	MAGA	Make America Great Again
	MbS	Muhammad bin Salman
	MERS	Middle East Respiratory Syndrome
	MSC	Munich Security Conference
	NIAID	National Institute of Allergy and Infectious Diseases
	NSA	National Security Agency
	NYSE	New York Stock Exchange
	OS	Operating system
	PFF	Progress and Freedom Foundation
	RCEP	Regional Comprehensive Economic Partnership
	RMA	Revolution in Military Affairs
	SCO	Shanghai Cooperation Organization
	SPV	Special Purpose Vehicles
	SWIFT	Society for Worldwide Interbank Financial Telecommunication
	TPP	Trans-Pacific Partnership
	UBI	Universal Basic Income
	WEF	World Economic Forum
	WHO	World Health Organization
	WMD	Weapon of mass destruction
	WTO	World Trade Organization

1. Introduction

All things are a flowing
Sage Heracleitus says;
But a tawdry cheapness
shall reign throughout our days.

                        Ezra Pound, *Hugh Selwyn Mauberley*

It seems, as one becomes older,
That the past has another pattern, and ceases to be a mere sequence –
Or even development: the latter a partial fallacy
Encouraged by superficial notions of evolution,
Which becomes, in popular mind, a means of disowning the past.
The moments of happiness—not the sense of well being,
Fruition, fulfillment, security or affection,
Or even a very good dinner, but the sudden illumination –
We had the experience but missed the meaning,
And approach to the meaning restores the experience
In a different form, beyond any meaning
We can assign to happiness. I have said before
That the past experience revived in the meaning
Is not the experience of one life only
But of many generations—not forgetting
Something that is probably quite ineffable:
The backward look behind the assurance
Of recorded history, the backward half-look
Over the shoulder, towards the primitive terror.

                   T.S. Eliot, *The Dry Salvages*, II, no. 3 of *Four Quartets*

The Raging Twenties started with a murder.

That lethality was amplified when a virus cannibalized virtually the whole planet, devouring time.

As time has been standing still—or imploded—ever since, we cannot even begin to imagine the consequences of the anthropological rupture caused by SARS-CoV-2.

A new world starts when language—either a living entity, or a virus from outer space (William Burroughs)—starts metastasizing new words.

A basket of concepts already stand out. Circuit breaker. Biosecurity. Negative feedback loops. State of exception. Necropolitics. New Brutalism. Hybrid Neofascism. And, as we shall see, New Viral Paradigm.

The proliferation of new words—and concepts—paradoxically developed in parallel with the slow fade out of The Word.

Cameroonian philosopher Achille Mbembe summed it all up: "This end of the word, this definitive triumph of the gesture and artificial organs over the word, the fact that the history of the word ends under our eyes, that for me is the historical development par excellence."

We all now live in Google town. Suddenly, we were forced to identify the lineaments of a new regime. A new mode of production: a turbo-capitalist survival engineered as Rentier Capitalism 2.0, where Silicon Valley behemoths take the place of estates, and also the State. That is the "techno-feudal" option, as defined by economist Cedric Durand.

Squeezed and intoxicated by information performing the role of a dominatrix, we were presented with a new map of Dystopia, packaged as a "new normal", featuring cognitive dissonance, a biosecurity paradigm, the inevitability of virtual work, social distancing as a political program, info-surveillance, and triumphant Trans-humanism.

A sanitary shock was superimposed over the economic shock—financialization always taking precedence over the real economy. But then the glimpse of a rosy future was offered towards more "inclusive" capitalism. A Great Reset. All thought out by a tiny plutocratic oligarchy, duly self-appointed as Saviors.

Baudrillard has shown us how sign value subsumes every other category—value, exchange-value, use-value. Our post-postmodern condition has gone way beyond the rule of signs. No more citizens: everyone now is collateral damage.

No wonder informed citizens started questioning whether they have been reduced to no more than victims of a full spectrum psy ops.

All of these themes evolve along the 25 small chapters of this book. And they also interact with the larger geopolitical chessboard. SARS-CoV-2 accelerated what was already a swing of the power center of the world towards Asia. The Empire we have been taught to accept as a fact of life is irretrievably losing its leadership position—and will have to deal with much pain implicit in the acceptance of an increasingly multipolar world.

Since WWII, most of the world lived as cogs of a tributary system, with the Empire constantly transferring wealth and influence to itself—via what analyst Ray McGovern describes as SS (security state) enforcing the will of the MICIMATT (Military-Industrial-Congressional-Intelligence-Media-Academia-Think-Tank) complex.

This world-system is fading out—especially due to the interpolations of the Russia-China strategic partnership. And that's the other overarching theme of this book.

To escape our excess hyper-reality show, what we need are Vanishing Points.

They can appear as trails—as in the Ho Chi Minh trail. Trails are rhizomes—configurations where there's no masterplan, but multiple entryways and multiple possibilities. No beginning and no end. As Gilles Deleuze described it, "the rhizome operates by variation, expansion, conquest, capture, offshoot."

Think of the chapters in this book as a series of rhizomes, networked to the narrative of a possible, emerging world-system in the essay titled *Eurasia, The Hegemon and the Three Sovereigns*.

In this running dialogue, Michel Foucault talks to Lao Tzu, Marcus Aurelius talks to Vladimir Putin, philosophy talks to geoeconomics—attempting to defuse the toxic interaction of the New Great Depression and variations of Cold War 2.0.

What happens overland is replicated overseas. We are all being carried forward through the tides by a harpooned whale, with no idea how, where, or when our journey ends. Like Melville's Ishmael, we've got to stay cool as we relentless fight the winds of fallacy, fiction, fraud and farce that the expiring system manipulates non-stop.

These columns, arranged chronologically, were originally published on *Asia Times*/Hong Kong, *Consortium News*/Washington D.C., and *Strategic Culture*/Moscow. They come from a global nomad. Since the mid-1990s I live between (mostly) East and West. With the exception of the first two months of 2020, I spent the bulk of the Raging Twenties in Asia, in Buddhist land.

So you will feel that the scent of these words is inevitably Buddhist, Taoist and Confucianist. In Asia we learn that the Tao transcends everything as it provides serenity. Talk about humanism without metaphysics.

That's quite the challenge—to fight Trans-humanism armed only with a method to achieve harmony and ban fear and angst. But what if we're able to muster our inner strength and choose a Taoist trail to ride the whale?

Bangkok, January 2021

2. IT'S THE US VS. RUSSIA-CHINA-IRAN

The Raging Twenties started with a bang with the targeted assassination of Maj. Gen. Qassem Soleimani.

Yet a bigger bang awaits us throughout the decade: the myriad declinations of the New Great Game in Eurasia, which pits the US against Russia, China and Iran, the three major nodes of Eurasia integration.

Every game-changing act in geopolitics and geoeconomics in the Raging Twenties will have to be analyzed in connection to this epic clash.

The Deep State and crucial sectors of the US ruling class are absolutely terrified that China is already outpacing the "indispensable nation" economically, and that Russia has outpaced it militarily.[1]

The Pentagon officially designates the three Eurasian nodes as "threats".

Hybrid War techniques—carrying inbuilt 24/7 demonization—will proliferate with the aim of containing China's "threat", Russian "aggression" and Iran's "sponsorship of terrorism". The myth of the "free market" will continue to drown under the imposition of a barrage of illegal sanctions, euphemistically defined as new trade "rules".

Yet that will be hardly enough to derail the Russia-China strategic partnership. To unlock the deeper meaning of this partnership, we need to understand that Beijing defines it as rolling towards a "new era". That implies strategic long-term planning—with the key date being 2049, the centennial of New China.

The horizon for the multiple projects of the Belt and Road Initiative (BRI)—as in the China-driven New Silk Roads—is indeed the 2040s, when Beijing expects to have fully woven a new,

---

[1] https://consortiumnews.com/2019/12/21/pepe-escobar-you-say-you-want-a-russian-revolution/

multipolar paradigm of sovereign nations/partners across Eurasia and beyond, all connected by an interlocking maze of belts and roads.

The Russian project– Greater Eurasia—somewhat mirrors BRI and will be integrated with it. BRI, the Eurasia Economic Union (EAEU), the Shanghai Cooperation Organization (SCO), the Asia Infrastructure Investment Bank (AIIB) are all converging towards the same vision.[2]

RUSSIA-CHINA PLAY REALPOLITIK

So this "new era", as defined by the Chinese, relies heavily on close Russia-China coordination, in every sector. Made in China 2025 is encompassing a series of techno/scientific breakthroughs. At the same time Russia has established itself as an unparalleled technological resource for weapons and systems that the Chinese still cannot match.

At the latest Brazil, Russia, India, China, and South Africa (BRICS) summit in Brasilia, President Xi Jinping told Vladimir Putin that "the current international situation with rising instability and uncertainty urge China and Russia to establish closer strategic coordination". Putin's response: "Under the current situation, the two sides should continue to maintain close strategic communication."

Russia is showing China how the West respects realpolitik power in any form, and Beijing is finally starting to use theirs. The result is that after five centuries of Western domination—which, incidentally, led to the decline of the Ancient Silk Roads—the Heartland is back, with a bang, asserting its preeminence.

On a personal note, my travels these past two years, from West Asia to Central Asia, and my conversations these past two months with analysts in Nur-Sultan, Moscow and Italy, have allowed me to get deeper into the intricacies of what sharp minds define as the Double Helix. We are all aware of the immense challenges ahead— while barely managing to track the stunning re-emergence of the Heartland in real time.

---

[2] https://onlinelibrary.wiley.com/doi/abs/10.1111/aspp.12497?af=R

In soft power terms, the sterling role of Russian diplomacy will become even more paramount—backed up by a Ministry of Defense led by Sergei Shoigu, a Turkophone Tuvan from Siberia, and an intel arm which is capable of constructive dialogue with everybody: India/Pakistan, North/South Korea, Iran/Saudi Arabia, Afghanistan.

This apparatus does smooth (complex) geopolitical issues over in a manner that still eludes Beijing.

In parallel, virtually the whole Asia-Pacific—from the Eastern Mediterranean to the Indian Ocean—now takes into full consideration Russia-China as a counter-force to US naval and financial overreach.

THE STAKES IN SOUTHWEST ASIA

The targeted assassination of Soleimani, for all its long-term fallout, is just one move in the Southwest Asia chessboard. What's ultimately at stake is a macro geoeconomic prize: a bridge from the Persian Gulf to the Eastern Mediterranean. [3]

Last summer, an Iran-Iraq-Syria trilateral established that "the goal of negotiations is to activate the Iranian-Iraqi-Syria load and transport corridor as part of a wider plan for reviving the Silk Road."

There could not be a more strategic connectivity corridor, capable of simultaneously interlinking with the International North South Transportation Corridor (INSTC); the Iran-Central Asia-China connection all the way to the Pacific; and projecting Latakia towards the Mediterranean and the Atlantic.

What's on the horizon is in fact a sub-sect of BRI in Southwest Asia. Iran is a key node of BRI; China will be heavily involved in the rebuilding of Syria; and Beijing-Baghdad signed multiple deals and set up an Iraqi-Chinese Reconstruction Fund (income from 300,000 barrels of oil a day in exchange for Chinese credit for Chinese companies rebuilding Iraqi infrastructure).

A quick look at the map reveals the "secret" of the US refusing

---

[3] https://schillerinstitute.com/blog/2020/01/13/iran-iraq-syria-plan-to-move-ahead-on-historic-transnational-land-bridge-railroad

to pack up and leave Iraq, as demanded by the Iraqi Parliament and Prime Minister: to prevent the emergence of this corridor by any means necessary. Especially when we see that all the roads that China is building across Central Asia—I navigated many of them in November and December—ultimately link China with Iran.

The final objective: to unite Shanghai to the Eastern Mediterranean—overland, across the Heartland.

As much as Gwadar port in the Arabian Sea is an essential node of the China-Pakistan Economic Corridor (CPEC), and part of China's multi-pronged "escape from Malacca" strategy, India also courted Iran to match Gwadar via the port of Chabahar in the Gulf of Oman.

So as much as Beijing wants to connect the Arabian Sea with Xinjiang, via CPEC, India wants to connect with Afghanistan and Central Asia via Iran.

Yet India's investments in Chabahar may come to nothing, with New Delhi still mulling whether to become an active part of the US "Indo-Pacific" strategy, which would imply dropping Tehran.

The Russia-China-Iran joint naval exercise in late December, starting exactly from Chabahar, was a timely wake-up to New Delhi. India simply cannot afford to ignore Iran and end up losing its key connectivity node, Chabahar.

The immutable fact; everyone needs and wants Iran connectivity. For obvious reasons; since the Persian empire this is the privileged hub for all Central Asian trade routes.

On top of it, Iran for China is a matter of national security. China is heavily invested in Iran's energy industry. All bilateral trade will be settled in yuan or in a basket of currencies bypassing the US dollar.

US neocons, meanwhile, still dream of what the Cheney regime was aiming at in the past decade; regime change in Iran leading to the US dominating the Caspian Sea as a springboard to Central Asia, only one step away from Xinjiang and weaponization of anti-China sentiment: a sort of New Silk Road in reverse to disrupt the Chinese vision.

THE BATTLE OF THE AGES

A new book, *The Impact of China's Belt and Road Initiative*, by Jeremy Garlick of the University of Economics in Prague, carries the merit of admitting that, "making sense of BRI is extremely difficult". [4]

This is an extremely serious attempt to theorize BRI's immense complexity—especially considering China's flexible, syncretic approach to policymaking, quite bewildering for Westerners. To reach his goal, Garlick gets into Tang Shiping's social evolution paradigm, delves into neo-Gramscian hegemony, and dissects the concept of "offensive mercantilism"—all that as part of an effort in "complex eclecticism".

The contrast with the pedestrian BRI demonization narrative emanating from US "analysts" is glaring. The book tackles in detail the multifaceted nature of BRI's trans-regionalism as an evolving, organic process.

Imperial policymakers won't bother to understand how and why BRI is setting a new global paradigm. The NATO summit in London last month offered a few pointers. NATO uncritically adopted three US priorities: even more aggressive policy towards Russia; containment of China (including military surveillance); and militarization of space—a spin-off the 2002 Full Spectrum Dominance doctrine.

So NATO will be drawn into the "Indo-Pacific" strategy—which means containment of China. And as NATO is the EU's weaponized arm, that implies the US interfering on how Europe does business with China—at every level.

Retired US Army Colonel Lawrence Wilkerson, Colin Powell's chief of staff from 2001 to 2005, cuts to the chase: "America exists today to make war. How else do we interpret 19 straight years of war and no end in sight? It's part of who we are. It's part of what the American Empire is. We are going to lie, cheat and steal, as Pompeo is doing right now, as Trump is doing right now, as Esper is doing right now (…) and a host of other members of my political party, the Republicans, are doing right now. We are going

---

[4] https://www.taylorfrancis.com/books/9781351182768

to lie, cheat and steal to do whatever it is we have to do to continue this war complex. That's the truth of it. And that's the agony of it."

Moscow, Beijing and Tehran are fully aware of the stakes. Diplomats and analysts are working on the trend, for the trio, to evolve a concerted effort to protect one another from all forms of Hybrid War—sanctions included—launched against each of them.

For the US, this is indeed an existential battle—against the whole Eurasia integration process, the New Silk Roads, the Russia-China strategic partnership, those Russian hypersonic weapons mixed with supple diplomacy, the profound disgust and revolt against US policies all across the Global South, the nearly inevitable collapse of the US dollar. What's certain is that the Empire won't go quietly into the night. We should all be ready for The Battle of the Ages.

Asia Times, January 2020

3. The Siren Call of a "System Leader"

A considerable spectrum of the liberal West takes the American interpretation of what civilization consists of to be something like an immutable law of nature. But what if this interpretation would be on the verge of an irreparable break down?

Michael Vlahos has argued that the US is not a mere nation-state but a "system leader"—"a civilizational power like Rome, Byzantium, and the Ottoman Empire."[5] And, we should add, China—which he did not mention. The system leader is "a universalistic identity framework tied to a state. This vantage is helpful because the United States clearly owns this identity framework today."

Intel stalwart Alastair Crooke, in a searing essay, digs deeper into how this "civilizational vision" was "forcefully unfurled across the globe" as the inevitable, American manifest destiny: not only politically—including all the accoutrements of Western individualism and neoliberalism—but coupled with "the metaphysics of Judeo-Christianity, too".[6]

Crooke also shows how deeply ingrained in the US elites is the notion that victory in the Cold War "spectacularly affirmed" the superiority of the US civilizational vision.

Well, the postmodern tragedy—from the point of view of US elites—is that soon this may not be the case anymore. The vicious civil war engulfing Washington for the past three years—with the whole world as stunned spectators—just accelerates the malaise.

Remember Pax Mongolica

It's sobering to consider that Pax Americana may be destined

---

[5] https://www.theamericanconservative.com/articles/the-rites-of-war/
[6] https://www.strategic-culture.org/news/2020/02/03/israel-in-the-middle-east-a-civilisational-and-metaphysical-war/

to a shorter historical existence than Pax Mongolica—established after Genghis Khan, as the head of a nomad nation, went about conquering the world.

Genghis first invested on a business/trade offensive to take over the Silk Roads, crushing the Kara-Kitais in Eastern Turkestan, conquering Islamic Khorezm, and annexing Bukhara, Samarkand, Bactria, Khorasan and Afghanistan. The Mongols reached the outskirts of Vienna in 1241 and the Adriatic Sea one year afterwards.

The superpower of the time extended from the Pacific to the Adriatic. We can barely imagine the shock for Western Christendom. Pope Gregory X was itching to know who were these conquerors of the world: perhaps they could be Christianized?

In parallel, only a victory by the Egyptian Mamluks in Galilee in 1260 saved Islam from being annexed to Pax Mongolica.

Pax Mongolica—a single, organized, efficient, tolerant power—coincided historically with the Golden Age of the Silk Roads. Kublai Khan—who lorded over Marco Polo—wanted to be more Chinese than the Chinese themselves. He wanted to prove that nomad conquerors turned sedentary could learn the rules of administration, commerce, literature and even navigation.

Yet when Kublai Khan died, the empire fragmented into rival khanates. Islam profited. Everything changed. A century later, the Mongols from China, Persia, Russia and Central Asia had nothing to do with their ancestors on horseback.

A jump cut to the young 21st century shows that the initiative, historically, is once again on the side of China, across the Heartland and lining up the Rimland. World-changing, game-changing enterprises don't originate in the West anymore—as has been the case from the 16th century up to the late 20th century.

For all the vicious wishful thinking that coronavirus will derail the "Chinese century", which will actually be the Eurasian Century, and amid the myopic tsunami of New Silk Roads demonization, it's always easy to forget that implementation of myriad projects has not even started.

It should be on 2021 that all those corridors/axes of continental development will pick up speed across Southeast Asia, the Indian

Ocean, Central Asia, Southwest Asia, Russia and Europe, in parallel to the Maritime Silk Road configuring a true Eurasian string of pearls from Dalian to Pireus, Trieste/Venice/Genoa and Hamburg/Rotterdam.

For the first time in two millennia, China is able to combine the dynamism of political and economic expansion both on the continental and maritime realms, something that the civilization-state did not experience since the short expeditionary stretch led by Admiral Zheng He in the Indian Ocean in the early 15th century. Eurasia, in the recent past, was under Western and Soviet colonization. Now it's going all-out multipolar—a series of complex, evolving permutations led by Russia-China-Iran-Turkey-India-Pakistan-Kazakhstan.

Every player has no illusions about the "system leader" obsessions: to prevent Eurasia from uniting under one power—or coalition (such as the Russia-China strategic partnership); make sure that Europe remains under US hegemony; prevent Southwest Asia—or the "Greater Middle East"—from being linked to Eurasian powers; and prevent by all means that Russia-China have unimpeded access to maritime lanes and trade corridors.

The message from Iran

In the meantime, a sneaking suspicion creeps in—that Iran's game plan, in an echo of Donbass in 2014, may be about sucking US neocons into a trademark Russian cauldron in case the regime change obsession is turbocharged.[7]

There is a serious possibility that under maximum pressure Tehran might eventually abandon the Joint Comprehensive Plan of Action (JCPOA) for good as well as the Treaty on the Non-Proliferation of Nuclear Weapons (NPT), thus openly inviting a US attack.

As it stands, Tehran has sent two very clear messages. The accuracy of the missile attack on the US Ayn Al-Asad base in Iraq, replying to the targeted assassination of Maj. Gen. Qassem Soleimani, means that any branch of the vast US Empire of Bases network is now vulnerable.

---

[7] https://tomluongo.me/2020/01/28/iran-russia-cauldron-neocons-podcast/

And the fog of non-denial denials surrounding the downing of the CIA Battlefield Airborne Communications Node (BACN)—essentially an aerial spook shop—in Ghazni, Afghanistan also carries a message.

CIA icon Mike d'Andrea, known as Ayatollah Mike, The Undertaker, the Dark Prince or all of the above, may or may not have been on board. Irrespective of the fact that no US government source will ever confirm or deny that Ayatollah Mike is dead or alive, or even that he exists at all, the message remains the same: your soldiers and spooks are also vulnerable.

Since Pearl Harbor no nation has dared to stare down the system leader so blatantly, as Iran did it in Iraq. Vlahos mentioned something I saw for myself in 2003, how "young American soldiers referred to Iraqis as 'Indians' as though Mesopotamia were the Wild West." Mesopotamia was one the crucial cradles of Civilization as we know it. Well, in the end those $2 trillion spent to bomb Iraq into democracy did no favors to the civilizational vision of the system leader.[8]

THE SIRENS AND LA DOLCE VITA

Now let's add aesthetics to our "civilizational" politics. Every time I visit Venice—which in itself is a living metaphor for both the flimsiness of empires and the Decline of the West—I retrace selected steps in *The Cantos*, Ezra Pound's epic masterpiece.

Last December, after many years, I went back to the church of Santa Maria dei Miracoli, also known as "the jewel box", which plays a starring role in The Cantos. As I arrived I told the custodian *signora* that I had come for "The Sirens". With a knowing smirk, she lighted my way along the nave to the central staircase. And there they were, sculpted on pillars on both sides of a balcony ("Crystal columns, acanthus, sirens in the pillar head", as we read in Canto 20).

These sirens were sculpted by Tullio and Antonio Lombardo,

---

[8] https://theconversation.com/the-iraq-war-has-cost-the-us-nearly-2-trillion-129617

sons of Pietro Lombardo, Venitian masters of the late 15th/early 16th century ("and Tullio Romano carved the sirens / as the old custode says: so that since / then no one has been able to carve them / for the jewel box, Santa Maria dei Miracoli", as we read in Canto 76).

Well, Pound misnamed the creator of the sirens. But that's not the point. The point is how Pound saw the sirens as the epitome of a strong culture ("the perception of a whole age, of whole congeries and sequence of causes, went into an assemblage of detail, whereof it wd. be impossible to speak in terms of magnitude", as Pound wrote in *Guide to Kulchur*).

As much as his beloved masterpieces by Giovanni Bellini and Piero della Francesca, Pound fully grasped how these sirens were the antithesis of *usura*—or the "art" of lending money at exorbitant interest rates, which not only deprives a culture of the best of art, as Pound describes it, but is also one of the pillars for the total financialization and marketization of life itself, a process that Pound brilliantly foresaw, when he wrote in *Hugh Selwyn Mauberley* that, "all things are a flowing / Sage Heracleitus says; /But a tawdry cheapness / shall reign throughout our days."

La Dolce Vita is turning 60 in 2020. Much as Pound's sirens, Fellini's now mythological tour de force in Rome is like a black and white celluloid palimpsest of a bygone era, the birth of the Swingin' Sixties. Marcello (Marcello Mastroianni) and Maddalena (Anouk Aimee), impossibly cool and chic, are like the Last Woman and the Last Man before the deluge of "tawdry cheapness". In the end, Fellini shows us Marcello despairing by the ugliness and, yes, cheapness intruding in his beautiful mini-universe—the lineaments of the trash culture fabricated and sold by the system leader about to engulf us all.

Pound was a human, all too human American maverick of unbridled classical genius. The system leader misinterpreted him; treated him as a traitor; caged him in Pisa; and dispatched him to a mental hospital in the US.[9] I still wonder whether he may have seen and appreciated La Dolce Vita during the 1960s, before he died in Venice in 1972. After all there was a little cinema within

---

[9] https://newrepublic.com/article/123283/case-ezra-pound

walking distance of the house in Calle Querini where he lived with Olga Rudge.

"Marcello!" We're still haunted by Anita Ekberg's iconic siren call half-immersed in the Fontana di Trevi. Today, still hostages of the crumbling civilizational vision of the system leader, at best we barely muster, as T.S. Eliot memorably wrote, a "backward half-look / over the shoulder / towards the primitive terror".

Asia Times, February 2020

4. THE WESTLESSNESS MYTH

Few postmodern political pantomimes have been more revealing than hundreds of so-called "international decision makers", mostly Western, wax lyric, disgusted or nostalgic over "Westlessness" at the Munich Security Conference (MSC).

"Westlessness" sounds like one of those constipated concepts issued from a post-party bad hangover at the Rive Gauche during the 1970s. In theory—but not French Theory—Westlessness in the age of Whatsapp should mean a deficit of multiparty action to address the most pressing threats to the "international order"—or (dis)order, as nationalism, derided as a narrow-minded populist wave, prevails.

Yet what Munich actually unveiled was some deep—Western—longing for those effervescent days of humanitarian imperialism, with nationalism in all its strands being cast as the villain impeding the relentless advance of profitable, neocolonial Forever Wars.

As much as the MSC organizers—a hefty Atlanticist bunch—tried to spin the discussions as emphasizing the need for multilateralism, a basket case of ills ranging from uncontrolled migration to "brain dead" NATO were billed as a direct consequence of "the rise of an illiberal and nationalist camp within the Western world". Like this was a rampage perpetrated by an all-powerful Hydra featuring Bannon-Bolsonaro-Orban heads.

Far from those West-is-More heads in Munich the courage to admit assorted nationalist counter-coups also qualify as blowback for the relentless Western plunder of the Global South via wars—hot, cold, financial, corporate-exploitative.

For what is worth, here's the MSC report.[10] Only two sentences would be enough to give away the MSC game: "In the post-Cold

---

[10] https://securityconference.org/assets/user_upload/MunichSecurity-Report2020.pdf'

War era, Western-led coalitions were free to intervene almost anywhere. Most of the time, there was support in the UN Security Council, and whenever a military intervention was launched, the West enjoyed almost uncontested freedom of military movement."

There you go. Those were the days when NATO, with full impunity, could bomb Serbia, miserably lose a war on Afghanistan, turn Libya into a militia hell and plot myriad interventions across the Global South. And of course none of that had any connection whatsoever with the bombed and the invaded forced into becoming refugees in Europe.

EAST IS EAST, WEST IS MORE

In Munich, South Korean Foreign Minister Kang Kyung-wha got closer to the point when she said she found "Westlessness" quite insular as a theme. She made sure to stress multilateralism is very much an Asian feature, expanding on the theme of Association of Southeast Asian Nations (ASEAN) centrality.

Russian Foreign Minister Sergey Lavrov, with his customary finesse, was sharper, noting how "the structure of the Cold War rivalry is being recreated" in Europe. Lavrov was a prodigy of euphemism while he noted how "escalating tensions, NATO's military infrastructure advancing to the East, exercises of unprecedented scope near the Russian borders, the pumping of defense budgets beyond measure—all this generates unpredictability."

Yet it was Chinese State Councilor and Foreign Minister Wang Yi who really got to the heart of the matter.[11] While stressing that, "strengthening global governance and international coordination is urgent right now", Wang said, "We need to get rid of the division of the East and the West and go beyond the difference between the South and the North, in a bid to build a community with a shared future for mankind."

"Community with a shared future" may be standard Beijing

11

https://www.youtube.com/watch?v=7YDdNg3nJG0&feature=youtu.be

terminology, but it does carry a profound meaning, as it embodies the Chinese concept of multilateralism as no single state having a priority and all nations sharing the same rights.

Wang went further: the West—with or without Westlessness—should get rid of its subconscious mentality of civilization supremacy; give up its bias against China; and "accept and welcome the development and revitalization of a nation from the East with a system different from that of the West." Wang is a sophisticated enough diplomat to know this is not going to happen.

Wang also could not fail to raise eyebrows among the Westlessness crowd to alarming levels when he stressed, once again, that the Russia-China strategic partnership will be deepened—alongside exploring "ways of peaceful coexistence" with the US and deeper cooperation with Europe.

What to expect from the so-called "system leader" in Munich was quite predictable.[12] And it was delivered, true to script, by current Pentagon head Mark Esper, yet another Washington revolving door practitioner.

THE TOP THREAT OF THE 21ST CENTURY

All Pentagon talking points were on display. China is nothing but a rising threat to the world order—as in "order" dictated by Washington. China steals Western know-how; intimidates all its smaller and weaker neighbors; seeks an "advantage by any means and at any cost."

As if any reminder to this well-informed audience was needed, China was once again placed at the top of the Pentagon's "threats", followed by Russia, "rogue states" Iran and North Korea, and "extremist groups". No one asked whether al-Qaeda in Syria is part of the list.

The "Communist Party and its associated organs, including the People's Liberation Army", were accused of "increasingly operating in theaters outside its borders, including Europe."

---

[12] https://www.asiatimes.com/2020/02/article/the-siren-call-of-a-system-leader/?_=2217007

Everyone knows only one "indispensable nation" is self-authorized to operate "in theaters outside its borders" to bomb others into democracy.

No wonder Wang was forced to qualify all of the above as "lies": "The root cause of all these problems and issues is that the US does not want to see the rapid development and rejuvenation of China, and still less would they want to accept the success of a socialist country."

So in the end Munich did disintegrate into the catfight that will dominate the rest of the century. With Europe de facto irrelevant and the EU subordinated to NATO's designs, Westlessness is indeed just an empty, constipated concept: all reality is conditioned by the toxic dynamics of China ascension and US decline.

The irrepressible Maria Zakharova once again nailed it: "They spoke about that country [China] as a threat to entire humankind.[13] They said that China's policy is the treat of the 21st century. I have a feeling that we are witnessing, through the speeches delivered at the Munich conference in particular, the revival of new colonial approaches, as though the West no longer thinks it shameful to reincarnate the spirit of colonialism by means of dividing people, nations and countries."

An absolute highlight of the MSC was when diplomat Fu Ying, the chairperson for the National People's Congress on Foreign Affairs, reduced Swamp Nancy Pelosi to dust with a simple question. [14]

Still, Secretary of State Mike "We Lie, We Cheat, We Steal" Pompeo was confident in Munich that "The West is winning." To which the Russia-China strategic partnership and myriad latitudes across the Global South might as well respond, "Bring it on".

Asia Times, February 2020

---

[13] https://tass.com/politics/1120699

[14] https://www.youtube.com/watch?v=taIYEG-HYx4&fbclid=IwAR03zt2V-Rt7FLGA3BcZBtMYiUFcTkwq9NVkV-006YZyVrHTKCbiumd8z8M

5. WE ARE ALL STOICS NOW

Earlier this week a delegation of Chinese medics arrived at Malpensa airport near Milan from Shanghai on a special China Eastern flight—carrying 400,000 masks and 17 tons of equipment. The salutation banner, in red and black, read, "We're waves from the same sea, leaves from the same tree, flowers from the same garden".

In a stance of supreme cross-cultural elegance, this was inspired by the poetics of Seneca, a Stoic. The impact, all over Italy, where people still study the classics, was immense.

For a 5,000-year-old civilization-state horrified when it must confront instances of *luan* ("chaos"), there's nothing more rejuvenating than post-chaos.

China is donating coronavirus test kits to Cambodia. China sent planeloads of masks, ventilators—and medics—to Italy and France.

China sent medics to Iran—under unilateral, illegal US sanctions—and Iraq—which the Pentagon is bombing again. China is helping across the (Eurasian) board—from the Philippines to Spain.

President Xi Jinping, in a phone call with Italy's Prime Minister Antonio Conte, pledged to establish a Health Silk Road in the wake of COVID-19, a companion to the New Silk Roads, or Belt and Road Initiative.

And then, there's the Philosophical Silk Road celebrated at an Italian airport, the meeting of Chinese and Greek/Latin Stoicism.

THE SLAVE, THE ORATOR AND THE EMPEROR

Stoicism, in Ancient Greece, was pop culture—reaching out in a way that the sophisticated Platonic and Aristotelian schools could only dream of. Like the Epicureans and the Skeptics, the Stoics owed a lot to Socrates—who always stressed that philosophy had to be practical, capable of changing our priorities in life.

The Stoics were very big on *ataraxia* (freedom of disturbance) as the ideal state of our mind. The wise man cannot possibly be troubled because the key to wisdom is knowing what not to care about.

So the Stoics were Socratic—in the sense that they were striving to offer peace of mind to Everyman. Like a Hellenistic version of the Tao.

The great ascetic Antisthenes was a companion of Socrates—and a precursor of the Stoics. The first Stoics took their name from the porch—*stoa*—in the Athenian market where official founder Zeno of Citium (333-262 BC) used to hang out. But the real deal was in fact Chrysippus, a philosopher specialized in logic and physics, who may have written no less than 705 books, none of which survived.

The West came to know the top Stoics as a Roman trio—Seneca, Epictetus and Marcus Aurelius. They are the role models of Stoicism as we know it today.

Epictetus (50-120 A.D.) was born as a slave in Rome, then moved to Greece, and spent his life always examining the nature of freedom.

Seneca (4-65 A.D.), a fabulous orator and decent dramatist, was exiled to Corsica when he was—falsely –accused of adultery with the sister of emperor Claudius. But afterwards he was brought back to Rome to educate the young Nero, and ended up sort of forced by Nero to commit suicide.

Marcus Aurelius, a humanist, was the prototypical reluctant emperor, living in a turbulent second century A.D. and configuring himself as a precursor of Schopenhaeur: Marcus saw life as really a drag.

Zeno's teachers were in fact Cynics—whose core intuition was that nothing mattered more than virtue. So the trappings of conventional society would have to be downgraded to the status of irrelevant distractions at best. No wonder there are very few true cynics left today.

It's enlightening to know that the upper classes of the Roman empire, their 1%, regarded Zeno's insights as quite solid, while—predictably—deriding the first punk in History, Diogenes the Cynic, who masturbated in the public square and carried a lantern trying to find a real man.

As much as for Heraclitus, for the Stoics a key element in the quest for peace of mind was learning how to live with the inevitable. This desire for serenity is one of their linkages with the Epicureans.

Stoics were adamant that most people have no clue about the universe they live in (imagine their reaction to social networks). Thus they end up confused in their attitudes towards life. In contrast to Plato and Aristotle, the Stoics were hardcore materialists. They would have none of that platonic "forms" talk in an ideal world: for the Stoics these were nothing but concepts in Plato's mind.

For the Epicureans, the world is the unplanned product of chaotic forces (tell that to Evangelist fanatics). The Stoics, in contrast, thought the world was a matter of organization down to the last detail.

For the Epicureans, the course of nature is not pre-determined: Fate intervenes in the form of random swerves of atoms. Fate, in Ancient Greece, actually meant Zeus. For the Stoics, everything happens according to Fate: an inexorable chain of cause and effect, developing in exact the same way again and again in a cycle of cosmic creation and destruction—a sort of precursor of Nietzsche's eternal recurrence.

It's All About Resigned Acceptance

The Stoics were heavily influenced by Heraclitus. Stoic physics dealt with the notion of interpenetration: the physical world as a stirred concoction of intermingled substances, quite an extraordinary precursor of the equivalence of energy and matter in Einstein.

What the postmodern world retains from the Stoics is the notion of resigned acceptance—which makes total sense if the world really works according to their insights. If Fate—once again, Zeus, not the Christian God—rules the world, and practically everything that happens is out of our hands, then realpolitik means to accept "everything to happen as it actually does happen", in the immortal words of Epictetus.

Thus it's pointless to get excited about stuff we cannot change. And it's pointless to be attached to things that we will eventually lose. But try selling this notion to the Masters of the Universe of financial capitalism.

So The Way—according to the Stoics—is to own only the essentials, and to travel light. Lao Tzu would approve it. After all anything we may lose is more or less gone already—thus we are already protected from the worst blows in life.

Perhaps the ultimate Stoic secret is the distinction by Epictetus between things that are under our control—our thoughts and desires—and what is not: our bodies, our families, our property, our lot in life, all elements that the expansion of COVID-19 now put in check.

What Epictetus tells us is that if we redirect our emotions to focus on what is in our power and ignore everything else, then "no one will ever be able to exert compulsion upon you, no one will hinder you—neither there's any harm that can touch you".

POWER IS ULTIMATELY IRRELEVANT

Seneca offered a definitive guide that we may apply to multiple strands of the 1%: "I deny that riches are a good, for if they were, they would make men good. As it is, since that which is found in the hands of the wicked cannot be called a good, I refuse to apply the term to riches."

The Stoics taught that to enter public life means to spread virtue and fight vice. It's a very serious business involving duty, discipline and self-control. This goes a long way to explain why over 70% of Italians now applaud the conduct of Prime Minister Conte in the fight against COVID-19. He did rise to the occasion, unexpectedly, as a neo-Stoic.

The Stoics regarded death as a useful reminder of one's fate—and the ultimate insignificance of the things of the world. Marcus Aurelius found enormous consolation in the shortness of life: "In a little while you will be no one and nowhere, even as Hadrian and Augustus are no more." When circumstances made it impossible to live up to the ideals of Stoic virtue, death was always a viable Plan B.

Epictetus also tells us we should not really be concerned about what happens to our body. Sometimes he seemed to regard death as the acceptable way out of any misfortune.

At the top of their game the Stoics made it clear that the difference between life and death was insignificant, compared to the difference between virtue and vice.

Thus the notion of a noble suicide. Stoic heroism is plain to see in the life and death of Cato The Younger as described by Plutarch. Cato was a fierce opponent of Caesar, and his integrity ruled the only possible way out was suicide.

According to Plutarch's legendary account, Cato, on his last night, defended a number of Stoic theses during dinner, retreated to his room to read Plato's *Phaedo*—in which, not by accident, Socrates argues that a true philosopher sees all of life as a preparation for death—and killed himself. Obviously he became a Stoic superstar for eternity.

The Stoics taught that wealth, status and power are ultimately irrelevant. Once again, Lao Tzu would approve. The only thing that can raise one man above others is superior virtue—of which everyone is capable, at least in principle. So yes, the Stoics believed we are all brothers and sisters. Seneca: "Nature made us relatives by creating us from the same materials and for the same destiny."

Imagine a system built on a selfless devotion to the welfare of others, and against all vanity. It's certainly not what inequality-provoking, financial turbo-capitalism is all about. Epictetus: "What ought one to say then as each hardship comes? I was practicing for this, I was training for this". Will COVID-19 show to a global wave of practicing neo-Stoics that there is another way?

Asia Times, March 2020

6. WHO PROFITS FROM THIS CONTROLLED DEMOLITION?

You don't need to read Foucault's work on biopolitics to understand that neoliberalism—in deep crisis since at least 2008—is a control/governing technique in which surveillance capitalism is deeply embedded. [15]

But now, with this world-system collapse—or controlled demolition—proceeding with breathtaking speed, neoliberalism is at a loss to deal with the next stage of dystopia, ever present in our hyper-connected angst: global mass unemployment.

Henry Kissinger, anointed oracle/gatekeeper of the ruling class, is predictably scared.[16] He claims that, "sustaining the public trust is crucial to social solidarity." He's convinced the Hegemon should "safeguard the principles of the liberal world order." Otherwise, "failure could set the world on fire."

That's so quaint. Public trust is dead across the spectrum. The liberal world "order" is now social Darwinist chaos. And just wait for the fire to rage.

The numbers are staggering. The Japan-based Asian Development Bank (ADB), in its annual economic report, may not have been exactly original. But it did note that the impact of the "worst pandemic in a century" will be as high as $4.1 trillion, or 4.8 percent of global gross domestic product (GDP).

And this an underestimation, as "supply disruptions, interrupted remittances, possible social and financial crises, and long-term effects on health care and education are excluded from the analysis."

We cannot even start to imagine the cataclysmic social consequences of the crash. Entire sub-sectors of the global

---

[15] https://www.palgrave.com/gp/book/9781403986559
[16] https://www.wsj.com/articles/the-coronavirus-pandemic-will-forever-alter-the-world-order

economy may not be recomposed at all.

The International Labour Organization (ILO) forecasts global unemployment at a conservative, extra 24.7 million people—hit especially in the aviation, tourism and hospitality industries.

The global aviation industry is a humongous $2.7 trillion business. That's 3.6% of global GDP. It employs 2.7 million people. Each one is responsible for creating another 24 jobs in air transport and tourism: everything from hotels and restaurants to theme parks and museums. That's a minimum of 65.5 million jobs around the world.

According to the ILO, income losses for workers may range from $860 billion to an astonishing $3.4 trillion. "Working poverty" will be the new normal—especially across the Global South.

"Working poor", in ILO terminology, means employed people living in households with a per capita income below the poverty line of $2 a day. As many as an additional 35 million people worldwide will become working poor in 2020.

Switching to feasible perspectives for global trade, it's enlightening to examine this report centered on the notorious hyperactive merchants and traders of Yiwu in eastern China—the world's busiest small-commodity business hub.[17]

Their experience spells out a long and difficult recovery. As the rest of the world is in a coma, Lu Ting, chief China economist at Nomura in Hong Kong stresses that China faces a 30% decline in external demand at least until next Fall.

Neoliberalism in reverse?

In the next stage, the strategic competition between the US and China will be no holds barred, as emerging narratives of China's new, multifaceted global role—on trade, technology, cyberspace, climate change—even more far-reaching than the New Silk Roads, will set in. That will also be the case in global public health policies. Get ready for an accelerated Hybrid War between the "Chinese

---

[17] https://www.caixinglobal.com/2020-04-06/in-depth-why-there-will-be-no-quick-cure-for-trade-after-the-pandemic-101539107.html

virus" narrative and the Health Silk Road.[18]

The latest report by the China Institute of International Studies would be quite helpful for the West—hubris permitting—to understand how Beijing adopted key measures putting the health and safety of the general population first.[19]

Now, as the Chinese economy slowly picks up, hordes of fund managers from across Asia are tracking everything from trips on the metro to noodle consumption to preview what kind of economy may be emerging post-lockdown.

In contrast, across the West, the prevailing doom and gloom elicited a priceless editorial from the FT.[20] Like James Brown in the 1980s Blues Brothers pop epic, the City of London seems to have seen the light or actually giving the impression it really means it. Neoliberalism in reverse. New social contract. "Secure" labor markets. Redistribution.

Cynics won't be fooled. The cryogenic state of the global economy spells out a vicious Great Depression 2.0 and an unemployment tsunami. The plebs eventually reaching for the pitchforks and the AR-15s en masse is now a distinct possibility. Might as well start throwing a few breadcrumbs to the beggars' banquet.

That may apply to European latitudes. The American story is in a class by itself.

For decades, we were led to believe that the world-system put in place after WWII provided the US with unrivalled structural power. Now, all that's left is structural fragility, grotesque inequalities, unpayable Himalayas of debt, and a rolling crisis.

No one is fooled anymore by the Fed's magic quantitative easing powers, or the acronym salad—TALF, ESF, SPV—inbuilt in the Fed/US Treasury exclusive obsession with big banks, corporations and the Goddess of the Market, to the detriment of the average American.

It was only a few months ago that a serious discussion evolved around the $2.5 quadrillion derivatives market imploding and

---

[18] https://asiatimes.com/2020/04/china-rolls-out-the-health-silk-road/
[19] https://share.weiyun.com/5YtIQm7
[20] https://www.ft.com/content/7eff769a-74dd-11ea-95fe-fcd274e920ca

collapsing the global economy, based on the oil price skyrocketing in case the Strait of Hormuz—for whatever reason—was shut down.

Now it's all about Great Depression 2.0: the whole system crashing as a result of the shutdown of the global economy. The question is absolutely legitimate: is the political and social cataclysm inbuilt in the global economic crisis arguably a larger catastrophe than COVID-19?

"Transparent" BlackRock

Wall Street, of course, lives in an alternative universe. In a nutshell, Wall Street turned the Fed into a hedge fund. The Fed is going to own at least two thirds of all US Treasury bills in the market before the end of 2020.

The US Treasury will be buying every security and loan in sight while the Fed will be the banker—financing the whole scheme.

So essentially this is a Fed/ Treasury merger. A behemoth dispensing loads of helicopter money.

And the winner is BlackRock—the biggest money manager on the planet, with tentacles everywhere, managing the assets of over 170 pension funds, banks, foundations, insurance companies, in fact a great deal of the money in private equity and hedge funds, everywhere. BlackRock—promising to be fully "transparent"—will buy all these securities and manage those dodgy SPVs on behalf of the Treasury.[21]

BlackRock, founded in 1988 by Larry Fink, may not be as big as Vanguard, but it's the top investor in Goldman Sachs, along with Vanguard and State Street, and with $6.5 trillion in assets, bigger than Goldman Sachs, JP Morgan and Deutsche Bank combined.

Now, BlackRock is the new operating system (OS) of Fed/Treasury.[22] The world's biggest shadow bank—and no, it's not

---

[21] https://www.ft.com/content/f3ea07b0-6f5e-11ea-89df-41bea055720b?fbclid=IwAR2QBBqUYiBUPW-zqAH5iQWDrAFeofT6Efr6IM8Ocb2E4xKAgbU6__wsHYw
[22] https://www.ft.com/content/08b897a5-aadb-40d7-922c-

Chinese.

It's not far-fetched to consider that BlackRock, with its multiple corporate tentacles, could easily set up, for instance, the mechanism of a national, digital ID in a flash.

Compared to this high-stakes game, mini-scandals such as the one around Georgia Senator Kelly Loeffler are peanuts.[23] Loeffler allegedly profited from inside information on COVID-19 by the Centers for Disease Control (CDC) to make a stock market killing. Loeffler is married to Jeffrey Sprecher—who happens to be the chairman of the New York Stock Exchange (NYSE), installed by Goldman Sachs.

While corporate media followed this story like headless chickens, post-COVID-19 plans, in Pentagon parlance, "move forward" by stealth.

The price? A meager $1,200 check per person for a month or two. Anyone knows that, based on median salary income, a typical American family would need $12,000 to survive for two months. Mnuchin, in an act of supreme affront, allows them a mere 10%. So American taxpayers will be left with a tsunami of debt while selected Wall Street players grab the whole loot, part of an unparalleled transfer of wealth upwards, complete with bankruptcies en masse of small and medium businesses.

Fink's letter to his shareholders almost gives the game away: "I believe we are on the edge of a fundamental reshaping of finance."[24]

And right on cue, he forecasted that, "in the near future—and sooner than most anticipate—there will be a significant reallocation of capital."

He was referring, then, to climate change. Now that refers to COVID-19.

431154ed968a?fbclid=IwAR1XRIwyLJegG7JK4DQElt2BU33cnOePm8 4syc-f3qwhnyRWz-zuc_THYuM

[23] https://www.huffpost.com/entry/kelly-loeffler-stock-scrutiny_n_5e851278c5b6f55ebf4788cc

[24] https://www.blackrock.com/corporate/investor-relations/larry-fink-ceo-letter

IMPLANT OUR NANOCHIP, OR ELSE

The game ahead will be focused on three elements: a social credit system, mandatory vaccination, and a digital currency.[25] This is what used to be called, according to the decades-old, time-tested CIA playbook, a "conspiracy theory". Well, it's actually happening.

A social credit system is something that China set up already in 2014. Before the end of 2020, every Chinese citizen will be assigned his/her own credit score—a de facto "dynamic profile", elaborated with extensive use of AI [Artificial Intelligence] and the internet of things (IoT), including ubiquitous facial recognition technology. This implies, of course, 24/7 surveillance, complete with Blade Runner-style roving robotic birds.

The US, the UK, France, Germany, Canada, Russia and India are not far behind. Germany, for instance, is tweaking its universal credit rating system, SCHUFA. France has an ID app very similar to the Chinese model, verified by facial recognition.

Mandatory vaccination is Bill "Malthus" Gates's wet dream, working in conjunction with the World Health Organization (WHO), the World Economic Forum (WEF) and Big Pharma.[26] He wants "billions of doses" to be enforced over the Global South.

Here it is, in his own words.[27] At 34:15: "Eventually what we'll have to have is certificates of who's a recovered person, who's a vaccinated person... Because you don't want people moving around the world where you'll have some countries that won't have it under control, sadly. You don't want to completely block off the ability for people to go there and come back and move around."

---

[25] https://www.crimeandpower.com/2020/01/05/one-world-digital-dictatorship/

[26] https://www.washingtonpost.com/opinions/bill-gates-heres-how-to-make-up-for-lost-time-on-covid-19/2020/03/31/ab5c3cf2-738c-11ea-85cb-8670579b863d_story.html?utm_campaign=wp_week_in_ideas&utm_medium=email&utm_source=newsletter&wpisrc=nl_idea

[27] https://www.youtube.com/watch?v=Xe8fIjxicoo

Then comes the last sentence which was erased from the official TED video. This was noted by Rosemary Frei, who has a master on molecular biology and is an independent investigative journalist in Canada. Gates says: "So eventually there will be this digital immunity proof that will help facilitate the global reopening up."

This "digital immunity proof" is crucial to keep in mind as the next steps take shape. We have reached full circle:[28] Event 201, WHO, Bill and Melinda Gates Foundation, mandatory vaccines, Big Pharma, ID2020.

The three top candidates to produce a coronavirus vaccine are American biotech firm Moderna, as well as Germans CureVac and BioNTech.[29] This mandatory vaccine carries the potential for the usual suspects of direct control over billions of people, in conjunction with an already extensively discussed Universal Basic Income (UBI) provided by a phantom state subordinated to financial powers.

Digital cash will be an offspring of blockchain. Not only the US,[30] but China and Russia are also interested in a national cryptocurrency. A global currency—of course controlled by central bankers—may soon be adopted in the form of a basket of currencies, and will circulate virtually. Endless permutations of the toxic cocktail of IoT, blockchain technology and the social credit system loom ahead.

So the key working hypothesis remains: this convulsion is a sophisticated global psyop, a global meltdown by design with COVID-19 used as cover for the usual suspects to bring in a new digital financial system and a mandatory vaccine—complete with a "digital identity" nanochip—embodying total control, and with no dissent allowed: what Slavoj Zizek calls the "erotic dream" of every totalitarian government.

Yet underneath it all, amid so much anxiety, a pent-up rage

---

[28] https://www.strategic-culture.org/news/2020/04/02/ground-control-planet-lockdown-only-test/
[29] https://mitsloan.mit.edu/ideas-made-to-matter/how-moderna-racing-to-a-coronavirus-vaccine
[30] https://www.sygna.io/blog/what-is-cryptocurrency-act-of-2020/"

seems to be gathering strength, to eventually explode in unforeseeable ways. As much as the system may be changing at breakneck speed, there's no guarantee even the 0.1% won't become road kill.

Consortium News, April 2020

7. GROUND CONTROL TO PLANET LOCKDOWN: THIS IS ONLY A TEST

As much as COVID-19 is a circuit breaker, a time bomb and an actual weapon of mass destruction (WMD), a fierce debate is raging worldwide on the wisdom of mass quarantine applied to entire cities, states and nations.

Those against it argue Planet Lockdown not only is not stopping the spread of COVID-19 but also has landed the global economy into a cryogenic state—with unforeseen, dire consequences. Thus quarantine should apply essentially to the population with the greatest risk of death: the elderly.

With Planet Lockdown transfixed by heart-breaking reports from the COVID-19 frontline, there's no question this is an incendiary assertion.

In parallel, a total corporate media takeover is implying that if the numbers do not substantially go down, Planet Lockdown—an euphemism for house arrest—remains, indefinitely.

Michael Levitt, 2013 Nobel Prize in chemistry and Stanford biophysicist, was spot on when he calculated that China would get through the worst of COVID-19 way before throngs of health experts believed, and that "What we need is to control the panic".[31]

Let's cross this over with some facts and dissident opinion, in the interest of fostering an informed debate.

The report *COVID-19—Navigating the Uncharted* was co-authored by Dr. Anthony Fauci—the White House face of the fight—, H. Clifford Lane, and CDC director Robert R. Redfield. So it comes from the heart of the US healthcare establishment.[32]

The report explicitly states, "the overall clinical consequences of COVID-19 may ultimately be more akin to those of a severe

---

[31] https://www.latimes.com/science/story/2020-03-22/coronavirus-outbreak-nobel-laureate
[32] https://www.nejm.org/doi/full/10.1056/NEJMe2002387

seasonal influenza (which has a case fatality rate of approximately 0.1%) or a pandemic influenza (similar to those in 1957 and 1968) rather than a disease similar to SARS or MERS, which have had case fatality rates of 9 to 10% and 36%, respectively."

On March 19, four days before Downing Street ordered the British lockdown, COVID-19 was downgraded from the status of "High Consequence Infectious Disease." [33]

John Lee, recently retired professor of pathology and former NHS consultant pathologist, has recently argued that, "the world's 18,944 coronavirus deaths represent 0.14 per cent of the total. These figures might shoot up but they are, right now, lower than other infectious diseases that we live with (such as flu)."[34]

He recommends, "a degree of social distancing should be maintained for a while, especially for the elderly and the immune-suppressed. But when drastic measures are introduced, they should be based on clear evidence. In the case of COVID-19, the evidence is not clear."

That's essentially the same point developed by a Russian military intel analyst. [35]

No less than 22 scientists—see here and here—have expanded on their doubts about the Western strategy. [36], [37]

Dr. Sucharit Bhakdi, Professor Emeritus of Medical Microbiology at the Johannes Gutenberg University in Mainz, has provoked immense controversy with an open letter to Chancellor Merkel, stressing the "truly unforeseeable consequences of the drastic containment measures which are currently being applied in large parts of Europe."

---

[33] https://www.gov.uk/guidance/high-consequence-infectious-diseases-hcid

[34] https://www.spectator.co.uk/article/The-evidence-on-COVID-19-is-not-as-clear-as-we-think

[35] https://www.fort-russ.com/2020/03/covid-19-it-may-turn-out-that-the-world-has-been-deceived-hints-russian-military-intelligence-agent/

[36] https://off-guardian.org/2020/03/24/12-experts-questioning-the-coronavirus-panic/"

[37] https://off-guardian.org/2020/03/28/10-more-experts-criticising-the-coronavirus-panic/

Even New York governor Andrew Cuomo admitted on the record about the error of quarantining elderly people with illnesses alongside the fit young population.

The absolutely key issue is how the West was caught completely unprepared for the spread of COVID-19—even after being provided a head start of two months by China, and having the time to study different successful strategies applied across Asia.

There are no secrets for the success of the South Korean model.

South Korea was producing test kits already in early January, and by March was testing 100,000 people a day, after establishing strict control of the whole population—to Western cries of "no protection of private life". That was before the West embarked on Planet Lockdown mode.

South Korea was all about testing early, often and safely—in tandem with quick, thorough contact tracing, isolation and surveillance.

COVID-19 carriers are monitored with the help of video-surveillance cameras, credit card purchases, smartphone records. Add to it SMS sent to everyone when a new case is detected near them or their place of work. Those in self-isolation need an app to be constantly monitored; non-compliance means a fine to the equivalent of $2,800.

CONTROLLED DEMOLITION IN EFFECT

In early March, the Chinese Journal of Infectious Diseases, hosted by the Shanghai Medical Association, pre-published an *Expert Consensus on Comprehensive Treatment of Coronavirus* in Shanghai.[38] Treatment recommendations included, "large doses of vitamin C...injected intravenously at a dose of 100 to 200 mg / kg per day. The duration of continuous use is to significantly improve the oxygenation index."

That's the reason why 50 tons of vitamin C was shipped to Hubei province in early February. It's a stark example of a simple "mitigation" solution capable of minimizing economic

---

[38] https://mp.weixin.qq.com/s/bF2YhJKiOfe1yimBc4XwOA

catastrophe.

In contrast, it's as if the brutally fast Chinese "people's war" counterpunch against COVID-19 had caught Washington totally unprepared. Steady intel rumbles on the Chinese net point to Beijing having already studied all plausible leads towards the origin of the SARS-Cov-2 virus—vital information that will be certainly weaponized, Sun Tzu style, at the right time.

As it stands, the sustainability of the complex Eurasian integration project has not been substantially compromised. As the EU has provided the whole planet with a graphic demonstration of its cluelessness and helplessness, every day the Russia-China strategic partnership gets stronger—increasingly investing in soft power and advancing a pan-Eurasia dialogue which includes, crucially, medical help.

Facing this process, the EU's top diplomat, Joseph Borrell, sounds indeed so helpless:[39] "There is a global battle of narratives going on in which timing is a crucial factor. [...] China has brought down local new infections to single figures—and it is now sending equipment and doctors to Europe, as others do as well. China is aggressively pushing the message that, unlike the US, it is a responsible and reliable partner. In the battle of narratives we have also seen attempts to discredit the EU (…) We must be aware there is a geopolitical component including a struggle for influence through spinning and the 'politics of generosity'. Armed with facts, we need to defend Europe against its detractors."

That takes us to really explosive territory. A critique of the Planet Lockdown strategy inevitably raises serious questions pointing to a controlled demolition of the global economy. What is already in stark effect are myriad declinations of martial law, severe social media policing in Ministry of Truth mode, and the return of strict border controls.

These are unequivocal markings of a massive social re-engineering project, complete with inbuilt full monitoring, population control and social distancing promoted as the new

---

[39] https://eeas.europa.eu/headquarters/headquarters-homepage/76379/coronavirus-pandemic-and-new-world-it-creating_en

normal.

That would be taking to the limit Secretary of State Mike "we lie, we cheat, we steal" Pompeo's assertion, on the record, that COVID-19 is a live military exercise: "This matter is going forward — we are in a live exercise here to get this right."

ALL HAIL BLACKROCK

So as we face a New Great Depression, steps leading to a Brave New World are already discernable. It goes way beyond a mere Bretton Woods 2.0, in the manner that Pam and Russ Martens superbly deconstruct the recent $2 trillion, Capitol Hill-approved stimulus to the US economy. [40]

Essentially, the Fed will "leverage the bill's $454 million bailout slush fund into $4.5 trillion".[41] And [42]no questions are allowed on who gets the money, because the bill simply cancels the Freedom of Information Act (FOIA) for the Fed.

The privileged private contractor for the slush fund is none other than BlackRock. Here's the extremely short version of the whole, astonishing scheme, masterfully detailed here. [43]

Wall Street has turned the Fed into a hedge fund. The Fed is going to own at least two thirds of all US Treasury bills wallowing in the market before the end of the year.

The US Treasury will be buying every security and loan in sight while the Fed will be the banker—financing the whole scheme.

So essentially this is a Fed/ Treasury merger. A behemoth dispensing loads of helicopter money—with BlackRock as the undisputable winner.

---

[40] https://wallstreetonparade.com/2020/03/stimulus-bill-allows-federal-reserve-to-conduct-meetings-in-secret-gives-fed-454-billion-slush-fund-for-wall-street-bailouts
[41] https://www.counterpunch.org/2020/03/30/washington-uses-the-pandemic-to-create-a-2-trillion-slush-fund-for-its-cronies/
[42] https://fashthenation.com/2020/03/how-trump-nationalized-u-s-financial-markets/
[43] https://fashthenation.com/2020/03/how-trump-nationalized-u-s-financial-markets/

BlackRock is widely known as the biggest money manager on the planet. Their tentacles are everywhere. They own 5% of Apple, 5% of Exxon Mobil, 6% of Google, second largest shareholder of AT&T (Turner, HBO, CNN, Warner Brothers)—these are just a few examples.

They will buy all these securities and manage those dodgy special Purpose Vehicles (SPVs) on behalf of the Treasury.

BlackRock not only is the top investor in Goldman Sachs. Better yet: Blackrock is bigger than Goldman Sachs, JP Morgan and Deutsche Bank combined. BlackRock is a serious Trump donor. Now, for all practical purposes, it will be the operating system—the Chrome, Firefox, Safari—of Fed/Treasury.

This represents the definitive Wall Street-ization of the Fed—with no evidence whatsoever it will lead to any improvement in the lives of the average American.

Western corporate media, en masse, have virtually ignored the myriad, devastating economic consequences of Planet Lockdown. Wall to wall coverage barely mentions the astonishing economic human wreckage already in effect—especially for the masses barely surviving, so far, in the informal economy.

For all practical purposes, the Global War on Terror (GWOT) has been replaced by the Global War on Virus (GWOV). But what is not being seriously analyzed is the Perfect Toxic Storm: a totally shattered economy; The Mother of All Financial Crashes—barely masked by the trillions in helicopter money from the Fed and the European Central Bank (ECB); the tens of millions of unemployed engendered by the New Great Depression; the millions of small businesses that will simply disappear; a widespread, global mental health crisis. Not to mention the masses of elderly, especially in the US, that will be issued an unspoken "drop dead" notice.

Beyond any rhetoric about "decoupling", the global economy is already, de facto, split in two. On one side, we have Eurasia, Africa and swathes of Latin America—what China will be painstakingly connecting and reconnecting via the New Silk Roads. On the other side, we have North America and selected Western vassals. A puzzled Europe lies in the middle.

A cryogenically induced global economy certainly facilitates a reboot. Trumpism is the New Exceptionalism—so that means an isolationist MAGA on steroids. In contrast, China will painstakingly reboot its market base along the New Silk Roads—Africa and Latin America included—to replace the 20% of trade/exports to be lost with the US.

The meager $1,200 checks promised to Americans are a de facto precursor of the much touted Universal Basic Income. They may become permanent as tens of millions of people will be permanently unemployed. That will facilitate the transition towards a totally automated, 24/7 economy run by AI—thus the importance of 5G.

And that's where ID2020 comes in.

AI AND ID2020

The European Commission is involved in a crucial but virtually unknown project, CREMA (Cloud Based Rapid Elastic Manufacturing) which aims to facilitate the widest possible implementation of AI in conjunction to the advent of a cashless One-World system.[44]

The end of cash necessarily implies a One-World government capable of dispensing—and controlling—UBI; a de facto full accomplishment of Foucault's studies on biopolitics. Anyone is liable to be erased from the system if an algorithm equals this individual with dissent.

It gets even sexier when absolute social control is promoted as an innocent vaccine.[45]

ID2020 is self-described as a benign alliance of "public-private partners".[46] Essentially, it is an electronic ID platform based on generalized vaccination. And its starts at birth; newborns will be provided with a "portable and persistent biometrically-linked digital identity."

---

[44] https://cordis.europa.eu/project/id/637066

[45] https://findbiometrics.com/new-id2020-project-to-build-biometric-id-program-around-infant-immunization

[46] https://euvsdisinfo.eu/report/the-coronavirus-moves-us-towards-a-totalitarian-state-of-the-world-and-the-introduction-of-agenda-id2020/"

GAVI, the Global Alliance for Vaccines and Immunization, pledges to "protect people's health" and provide "immunization for all".[47] Top partners and sponsors, apart from the WHO, include, predictably, Big Pharma.

At the ID2020 Alliance summit last September in New York, it was decided that the "Rising to the Good ID Challenge" program would be launched in 2020. That was confirmed by the World Economic Forum this past January in Davos. The digital identity will be tested with the government of Bangladesh.

That poses a serious question: was ID2020 timed to coincide with what a crucial sponsor, the WHO, qualified as a pandemic? Or was a pandemic absolutely crucial to justify the launch of ID2020?

As game-changing trial runs go, nothing of course beats Event 201, which took place less than a month after ID2020. [48]

The Johns Hopkins Center for Health Security in partnership with, once again, the WEF, as well as the Bill and Melinda Gates Foundation, described Event 201 as "a high-level pandemic exercise". The exercise "illustrated areas where public/private partnerships will be necessary during the response to a severe pandemic in order to diminish large-scale economic and societal consequences."

With COVID-19 in effect as a pandemic, the Johns Hopkins Bloomberg School of Public Health was forced to issue a statement basically saying they just "modeled a fictional coronavirus pandemic, but we explicitly stated that it was not a prediction". [49]

There's no question "a severe pandemic, which becomes 'Event 201' would require reliable cooperation among several industries, national governments, and key international institutions", as spun by the sponsors. COVID-19 is eliciting exactly this kind of "cooperation". Whether it's "reliable" is open to endless debate.

The fact is that, all over Planet Lockdown, a groundswell of public opinion is leaning towards defining the current state of

---

[47] https://www.gavi.org
[48] http://www.centerforhealthsecurity.org/event201/
[49] http://www.centerforhealthsecurity.org/newsroom/center-news/2020-01-24-Statement-of-Clarification-Event201.htm

affairs as a global psyop: a deliberate global meltdown—the New Great Depression—imposed on unsuspecting citizens by design.

The powers that be, taking their cue from the tried and tested, decades-old CIA playbook, of course are breathlessly calling it a "conspiracy theory". Yet what vast swathes of global public opinion observe is a—dangerous—virus being used as cover for the advent of a new, digital financial system, complete with a forced vaccine cum nanochip creating a full, individual, digital identity.

The most plausible scenario for our immediate future reads like clusters of smart cities linked by AI, with people monitored full time and duly micro-chipped doing what they need with a unified digital currency, in an atmosphere of Bentham's and Foucault's Panopticon on overdrive.

So if this is really our future, the existing world-system has to go. This is a test, this is only a test.

Strategic Culture, April 2020

8. HOW THE RIDDLER MAY TEACH US TO FIGHT A DISEASE

He was known as "The Riddler". Even "The Dark". Heraclitus of Ephesus was one of a kind.

In his heart of hearts a contemptuous aristocrat, this master of paradox despised all so-called wise men and the mobs that adored them. Heraclitus was the definitive precursor of social distancing.

We, unfortunately, owe the "pre-Socratic" reductionist label to 19th century historians, who sold to modernity the notion that these thinkers were not so preeminent because they lived before Socrates (469-399 BC) throughout the 6th and 5th century BC, in assorted latitudes found in today's Greece, Italy and Turkey.

Yet Nietzsche nailed it: the pre-Socratics invented all the archetypes of all the history of philosophy. And if that was not enough, they invented science as well. Their Grandmaster Flash was, unequivocally, Heraclitus.

Nature as a perpetual detective story

Only around 130 fragments of Heraclitus thinking managed to survive—prefiguring Walter Benjamin's intuition that the beauty of knowledge is encapsulated by the fragment.

Let's start with "Nature loves to hide". Heraclitus established that Nature—and the world—are ambiguous par excellence, in a never- ending film noir. As Nature is a nest of riddles, he could only use riddles to examine it.

It's tempting to imagine Heraclitus as a doppelganger of the famous Delphic oracle, which "neither declares nor conceals, but gives a sign". He's certainly a precursor of Twin Peaks (the owls are not what they seem)[50]. Legend has it that the only copy of his book was consigned to a temple in Ephesus in the early 5th century BC, shortly after the death of Pythagoras, so the mobs wouldn't have access to it. Heraclitus, a member of the Ephesus

---

[50] https://www.youtube.com/watch?v=mbi7rq-TSk8"

royal family, would not have settled for less.

So we, as a race, are essentially a misguided bunch. "Men are deceived in the recognition of what is obvious, like Homer who was wisest of all the Greeks". Heraclitus compared our lot to beasts, winos, deep sleepers and even children—as in our opinions are like toys. We are incapable of grasping the true *logos*. History, with rare exceptions, seems to have vindicated him.

There are two key Heraclitus mantras.

1) "All things come to pass according to conflict". So the basis of everything is turmoil. Everything is in flux. Life is a battleground (Sun Tzu would approve it).

2) "All things are one". This means opposites attract. This is what Heraclitus found when he went tripping inside his soul—with no help of lysergic substances. No wonder he faced a Sisyphean task trying to explain this to us, mere children.

And that brings us to the river metaphor. Everything in nature depends on underlying change. Thus, for Heraclitus, "as they step into the same rivers, other and still other waters flow upon them". So each river is composed of ever-changing waters.

If you step into the Ganges or the Amazon one day, that would be something completely different compared to another day.

Thus the notorious mantra *Panta rhei* ("everything flows"). Flux and stability, unity and diversity, are like night and day.

One river may consist of many waters, and even if there are many waters, it's still one river. That's how Heraclitus reconciled conflict and unity into harmony—quite an Eastern philosophy concept.

No fragment tells it explicitly. But what's fascinating is that flux in unity—and unity in flux—do look like moving parts of the *logos*, the guiding principle of the world, which no one before him had managed to understand.

Let me stand next to your fire

Everything flows. And that brings us to war—and once again Heraclitus meets Sun Tzu: "War is father of all and king of all".

That also brings us to fire. The world is "fire ever living" and "fire for all things, as goods for gold and gold for goods". Here Heraclitus seems to be equating gold as a vehicle of economic exchange to fire as a vehicle of physical change. He would have despised fiat money; Heraclitus was definitely in favor of the gold standard.

No wonder Heraclitus fascinated Nietzsche because he was essentially proposing a cyclical theory of the universe—Nietzsche's eternal recurrence—with everything turning into fire in serial cosmic bust-ups.

Heraclitus was a Taoist and a Buddhist. If opposites are ultimately the same, this implies the unity of all things.

Heraclitus even foresaw the reaction we should have towards COVID-19: "It is disease that makes health sweet and good, hunger satiety, weariness rest." The Tao would approve it. In the Heraclitus framework of serial cosmic recycling, disease gives health its full significance.

This collective attitude could go a long way to explain the relative success of Eastern societies in the fight against COVID-19 compared to the West.

And once again, all this Heraclitean interconnectivity could not be more Eastern—from Tao to Buddhism. No wonder the grandmasters of Western civilization, Plato and Aristotle, did not exactly get it.

Plato distorted Heraclitus because he based his analysis on Cratylus, a philosopher who misunderstood Heraclitus in the first place. Because Plato and Aristotle basically regurgitated his reductionist interpretation, everyone afterwards followed them, and not the Original Riddler.

For Plato and Aristotle, it was impossible to understand Heraclitus because they seemed to have taken "you cannot step into the same river twice" literally.

Heraclitus in fact discovered, for all humanity to see, that rivers—and everything else in nature—are constantly changing, they're all about flux, even when they seem still. Call that a definition of History.

At least Plato's misguided interpretation raised a key question we are still debating 2,500 years later: how is it possible to have certain knowledge of an ever-changing world? Or as Nietzsche famously put it: there are no facts, only interpretations.

So because of Plato's misunderstanding, Heraclitus the genuine article became a sideshow in the history of thought. The

Riddler would not have given a damn. It's up to us to do him justice in these anguished times.

Asia Times, April 2020

9. TOTAL SYSTEM FAILURE OR THE BIRTH OF A NEW ECONOMY?

Nobody, anywhere, could have predicted what we are now witnessing, in a matter of only a few weeks: the accumulated collapse of global supply chains, aggregate demand, consumption, investment, exports, mobility.

Nobody is betting on an "L" recovery anymore—not to mention "V". Any projection for global GDP in 2020 gets into falling off a cliff territory.

In industrialized economies, where roughly 70% of the workforce is in services, countless businesses in myriad industries won't recover, forecasting a rolling financial collapse that will eclipse the Great Depression.

That spans the whole spectrum of possibly 47 million US workers soon to be laid off, with the unemployment rate skyrocketing to 32%, all the way to Oxfam warning that by the time the pandemic is over half of the world's population of 7.8 billion people could be living in poverty.

According to the World Trade Organization (WTO)'s most optimistic 2020 scenario—certainly to become outdated before the end of Spring—global trade would shrink by 13%.

This is a sobering, Asia-centered analysis on what lies ahead for global trade.[51] A more realistic, gloomier, WTO scenario sees global trade plunging by 32%.

What we are witnessing is not only a massive globalization short circuit: it's a cerebral shock extended to hyperconnected, simultaneously confined 3 billion people. Their bodies may be blocked, but as electromagnetic beings, their brains keep working –with possible, unforeseen (political) consequences.

Soon we will be facing three major, interlocking debates: the

---

[51] https://www.caixinglobal.com/2020-04-06/in-depth-why-there-will-be-no-quick-cure-for-trade-after-the-pandemic-101539107.html

management of the crisis, in many cases appalling; the search for future models; and the reconfiguration of the world-system.

This is just a first approach in what should be seen as a do-or-die cognitive competition.

WATCH THE PARTICLE ACCELERATOR

Sound analyses of what could be the next economic model are already popping up.[52] As background, a really serious debunking of all (dying) neoliberalism development myths can be seen here.[53]

Yes, a new economic model should be revolving around these axes: AI computing; automated manufacturing; solar and wind energy; high-speed data transfer—as in 5G; and nanotechnology.

China, Japan, South Korea, Taiwan are very well positioned for what's ahead, as well as selected European latitudes.

Plamen Tonchev, head of Asia unit at the Institute of International Economic Relations in Athens, points to the possible reorganization—short term—of Belt and Road Initiative (BRI) projects, privileging investment in energy, export of solar panels, 5G networks and the Health Silk Road. .[54],[55]

COVID-19 is like a particle accelerator—consolidating tendencies that were already developing. China had already demonstrated—for the whole planet to see—that economic development, under a control system, has nothing to do with Western liberal democracy.

On the pandemic, China demonstrated—also for the whole planet to see—that imposing controls the West derided as "draconian" and "authoritarian", coupled with a strategic scientific approach (profusion of test kits, protection equipment,

---

[52] ttps://www.nakedcapitalism.com/2020/04/the-coronavirus-pandemic-has-opened-the-curtains-on-the-worlds-next-economic-model.html

[53] https://www.youtube.com/watch?v=pBXRWh2US84&feature=youtu.be

[54] https://thediplomat.com/2020/04/the-belt-and-road-after-covid-19/

[55] https://asiatimes.com/2020/04/china-rolls-out-the-health-silk-road/

ventilators, experimental treatments), containment of COVID-19 is possible.

This is already translating into incalculable soft power—which will be exercised along the Health Silk Road. Trends seem to point to China strategically reinforced all along the spectrum—especially in the Global South. China is playing go, weiqi. Stones will be taken from the geopolitical board.

SYSTEM FAILURE WELCOMED?

In contrast, Western banking and finance scenarios could not be gloomier. As this Britain-centric analysis argues, "it is not just Europe. Banks may not be strong enough to fulfill their new role as saviors in any part of the world, including the US, China, and Japan. None of the major lending systems were ever stress-tested for an economic deep freeze lasting months."[56]

So "the global financial system will crack under the strain", with a by now quite possible "pandemic shutdown lasting more than three months" capable of causing "economic and financial 'system failure'".

As system failures go, nothing remotely approaches the possibility of a quadrillion dollar derivative implosion. I've addressed the derivatives story on Asia Times for quite a while because this is a real nuclear issue.

Capital One is number 11 on the list of the largest banks in the US by assets. They are already in deep trouble on their derivative exposures. As my New York sources told me, Capital One made a terrible trade, betting via derivatives that oil would not plunge to where it is now—17-year lows.

Mega pressure is on all those Wall Street outfits that gave oil companies the equivalent of puts on all their oil production at prices above $50.00 a barrel. These puts now come due—and the strain on the Wall Street houses and US banks will become unbearable.

This is just the beginning, and is bound to get much worse.

---

[56] https://www.telegraph.co.uk/business/2020/04/07/world-banking-system-cannot-weather-long-lockdown/

Imagine most of US industry being shut down. Corporations—like Boeing, for instance—are going to go bankrupt. Bank loans to these corporations will be wiped out. As these loans are wiped out, the banks are going to get in major trouble.

Wall Street, totally linked to the derivative markets, will feel the pressure of the collapsing American economy. The Fed bailout of Wall Street will start coming apart. Talk about a—nuclear—chain reaction.

Once again, in a nutshell: The Fed has lost control of the money supply in the US. Banks can now create unlimited credit from their base—and that sets up the US for potential hyperinflation if the money supply grows non-stop and production collapses—as it is collapsing right now because the economy is in shutdown mode.

If derivatives start to implode, the only solution for all major banks in the world will be immediate nationalization—much to the ire of the Goddess of the Market. Deutsche Bank—in major trouble—has a 7 trillion euro derivatives exposure, twice the annual GDP of Germany.

No wonder New York business circles are absolutely terrified. They insist that if the US does not immediately go back to work, and these possibly quadrillions of dollars of derivatives start to rapidly implode, the economic crises that will unfold will create such a collapse the magnitude of which has not been witnessed in history, with incalculable consequences.

Or perhaps this will be just the larger than life spark to start a new economy.

Asia Times, April 2020

10. HOW CONFUCIUS, BUDDHA AND THE TAO ARE WINNING THIS "WAR"

As the Raging Twenties unleash a radical reconfiguration of the planet, coronavirus (literally "crowned poison") has for all practical purposes served a poisoned chalice of fear and panic to myriad, mostly Western, latitudes.

Berlin-based South Korean philosopher Byung-Chul Han has forcefully argued the victors are the "Asian states like Japan, Korea, China, Hong Kong, Taiwan or Singapore that have an authoritarian mentality which comes from their cultural tradition [of] Confucianism. People are less rebellious and more obedient than in Europe. They trust the state more. Daily life is much more organized. Above all, to confront the virus Asians are strongly committed to digital surveillance. The epidemics in Asia are fought not only by virologists and epidemiologists, but also computer scientists and big data specialists."[57]

That's a reductionist view—and plenty of nuance should apply. Take South Korea—which is not "authoritarian", rather as democratic as top Western liberal powers. What we had in a nutshell was the civic mindedness of the overwhelming majority of the population reacting to sound, competent government policies.

Seoul went for fast mobilization of scientific expertise; immediate massive testing; extensive contact tracing; and social distancing as well—but crucially, most of it voluntary, not imposed by the central power. Because these moves were organically integrated, South Korea did not need drastic restriction of movement and to close down airports.

Hong Kong's success is due in large part to a superb health care

---

[57] https://elpais.com/ideas/2020-03-21/la-emergencia-viral-y-el-mundo-de-manana-byung-chul-han-el-filosofo-surcoreano-que-piensa-desde-berlin.html

system where people in the frontline—with institutional memory of recent epidemics such as SARS—were willing to go on strike if serious measures were not adopted. Hong Kong and Taiwan's success was also due in large part to myriad professional links between their healthcare and public health systems.

BARBARISM WITH A HUMAN FACE

Then there's Big Data. Byung-Chul-Han argues that neither in China or other Asian nations there's enough critical analysis in relation to digital vigilance and Big Data—and that also has to do with culture, because Asia is about collectivism, and individualism is not on the forefront.

Well, that's way more nuanced. Across Asia, digital progress is pragmatically evaluated in terms of effectiveness. Wuhan deployed Big Data via thousands of investigative teams, searching for possibly infected individuals, and choosing who had to be under observation and who had to be quarantined. Borrowing from Foucault, we can call it digital biopolitics.

Where Han is correct is when he says that the pandemic may redefine the concept of sovereignty: "The sovereign is the one who resorts to data. When Europe proclaims a state of alarm or closes borders, it's still chained to old models of sovereignty."

The response across the EU, including especially the European Commission in Brussels, has been appalling, with glaring evidence of powerlessness and lack of any serious preparations—even given a head start of many weeks by what was developing in China.

The first instinct was—what else—to close borders; hoard whatever puny equipment was available; and, then, social Darwinism style, it was every nation for itself, with battered Italy left totally to itself.

This is a relatively decent summary of the disaster in France. [58]

The severity of the crisis especially in Italy and Spain—with elders left to die to the "benefit" of the young—was due to a very specific EU political economy choice: the austerity diktat imposed

---

[58] https://www.mediapart.fr/journal/france/110420/covid-19-chronologie-d-une-debacle-francaise

across the eurozone. It's as if, in a macabre way, Italy and Spain are paying literally in blood to remain part of a currency, the euro, which they should never have adopted in the first place.

Going forward, Slavoj Zizek gloomily predicts for the West "a new barbarism with a human face—ruthless survivalist measures enforced with regret and even sympathy, but legitimized by expert opinions".

In contrast, Han predicts, China will now be able to sell its digital police state as a model of success against the pandemic. China will display the superiority of its system even more proudly."

Alexander Dugin ventures way beyond anyone else. He's already conceptualizing the notion of a state in mutation (like the virus) turning into a "military-medical dictatorship", just as we're witnessing the collapse of the global liberal world in real time. [59]

ENTER THE TRIAD

I offer as a working hypothesis that the Asia triad of Confucius, Buddha and Lao Tzu has been absolutely essential in shaping the perception and serene response of hundreds of millions of people across various Asian nations to COVID-19—compared to the prevalent fear, panic and hysteria mostly fed by corporate media across the West.

The Tao ("the way") as configured by Lao Tzu is about how to live in harmony with the world. Being confined necessarily leads to delving into yin instead of yang; slowing down; and embarking on a great deal of reflection.

Yes, it's all about culture—but culture rooted in ancient philosophy, and practiced in everyday life. That's how we can see *wu wei*—"action of non-action"—applied to how to deal with a quarantine. "Action of non-action" means action without intent. Rather than fighting against the vicissitudes of life, as in confronting a pandemic, we should allow things to take their natural course.

---

[59] https://www.geopolitica.ru/en/article/pandemic-and-politics-survival-horizons-new-type-dictatorship"

That's much easier when we know that the Tao teaches, "health is the greatest possession. Contentment is the greatest treasure. Confidence is the greatest friend. Non-being is the greatest joy."

It also helps to know that "life is a series of natural and spontaneous choices. Don't resist them—that only creates sorrow. Let reality be reality. Let things flow naturally forward in whatever way they like."

Buddhism runs in parallel to the Tao: "All conditioned things are impermanent—when one sees this with wisdom, one turns away from suffering."

And to keep our vicissitudes in perspective, it helps to know that,

"better it is to live one day seeing the rise and fall of things than to live a hundred years without ever seeing the rise and fall of things."

As far as keeping much needed perspective, nothing beats, "the root of suffering is attachment."

And then, there's the ultimate perspective: "Some do not understand that we must die. But those who do realize this settle their quarrels."

Confucius has been an overarching presence across the COVID-19 frontline, as an astonishing 700 million Chinese citizens were kept for weeks under different forms of quarantine.

We can easily imagine them clinging to a few pearls of wisdom, such as "death and life have their determined appointments; riches and honors depend upon heaven". Or "he who learns but does not think, is lost. He who thinks but does not learn is in great danger."

Most of all, in an hour of extreme turbulence, it brings comfort to know that, "the strength of a nation derives from the integrity of the home."

And in terms of fighting a dangerous and invisible enemy on the ground, it helps to know that "when it is obvious that the goals cannot be reached, don't adjust the goals, adjust the action steps."

So what would be the ultimate insight a serene East can offer to the West in such hard times? It's so simple, and it's all in the Tao: "From caring comes courage."

Asia Times, April 2020

11. THE CITY IN A TIME OF PLAGUE

> "The plague-stricken town, traversed throughout with hierarchy, surveillance, observation, writing; the town immobilized by the functioning of an extensive power that bears in a distinct way over all individual bodies—this is the utopia of the perfectly governed city."
>
> Michel Foucault, *Discipline and Punish*

Predictably eyeing the Decline and Fall of the American Empire, a serious academic debate is raging around the working hypothesis of historian Kyle Harper, according to whom viruses and pandemics—especially the Justinian plague in the 6th century—led to the end of the Roman Empire. [60], [61]

Well, history actually teaches us that epidemics are revelatory moments as much as social transformers.

Patrick Boucheron, a crack historian and a professor at the esteemed College de France, offers a very interesting perspective.[62] Incidentally, before the onset of COVID-19, he was about to start a seminar on the Black Death medieval plague.

Boucheron's view of Boccaccio's *Decameron*, written in 1350 and about young Florentine aristocrats who fled to the Tuscan countryside to tell stories, focuses on the plague's character as a "horrible beginning" that tears apart social liaisons, provokes a funerary panic and has everyone wallowing in anomie.

Then he draws a historical parallel with Thucydides writing

---

[60] https://www.amazon.com/gp/product/B071SLPWVL/ref=dbs_a_def-_rwt_hsch_vapi_tkin_p1_i0

[61] https://www.medievalists.net/2019/11/the-plague-of-justinian-may-not-have-that-devastating-researchers-suggest/

[62] ttps://www.mediapart.fr/journal/culture-idees/120420/patrick-boucheron-en-quoi-aujourd-hui-differe-d-hier?page_article=3

about the Athens plague in the summer of 430 BC[63] Pushing it to the limit, we may venture that Western literature actually starts with a plague—described in Book one of the Iliad by Homer.[64]

Thucydides' description of the Great Plague—actually typhoid fever—is a literary tour de force as well. In our current setting, that's more relevant than the "Thucydides trap" controversy—as it's idle to compare the context in ancient Athens with the current US-China Hybrid War.

Both Socrates and Thucydides, incidentally, survived the plague. They were tough, and acquired immunity from their earlier exposure to typhoid. Pericles, the leading citizen of Athens, was not so lucky: he died at 66, a victim of the plague.

THE CITY IN FEAR

Boucheron wrote an immensely interesting book, *Conjurer la Peur* ("To Conjure Fear") telling the story of Siena a few years before the Black Death, in 1338.[65] This is the Siena pictured by Ambrogio Lorenzetti in the walls of the Palazzo Pubblico—one of most spectacular allegorical frescoes in History.

In his book, Boucheron writes about political fear before it is engulfed by biological fear. Nothing could be more contemporary.

In Lorenzetti's Allegory of Bad Government, the court of bad justice is governed by a devil holding a poisoned chalice (today that would be the "crowned poison"—or coronavirus). The devil's eyes are crossed and one of his feet is over a goat's horns. Floating above his head we find Avarice, Pride, and Vainglory (match them with contemporary political "leaders"). War, Treason, and Fury sit to his left (the US Deep State?) and Discord, Fraud, and Cruelty on his right (casino capitalist financialization?) Justice is bound, and her scales have fallen: talk about an allegory of the

---

[63] https://www.livius.org/sources/content/thucydides-historian/the-plague/
[64] https://www.poetryintranslation.com/PITBR/Greek/Iliad1.php
[65] https://www.amazon.com/Conjurer-peur-Sienne-1338-politique/dp/2021134997/ref=sr_1_1?dchild=1&keywords=Conjurer+la+Peur+Patrick+Boucheron&qid=1587096485&s=digital-text&sr=8-1

"international community".

Boucheron pays special attention to the city as depicted by Lorenzetti -- That's the city at war—compared to the harmonious city in the *Allegory of Good Government*.[66] The crucial point is that this is a depopulated city—much as our cities in quarantine now. Only men in arms are circulating, and as Boucheron tells it, "we guess that behind the walls, people are dying". So this image has not changed today—deserted streets, quite a few elderly people dying in silence at their homes.

Boucheron then makes a startling connection with the frontispiece of Hobbes' *Leviathan*, published in 1651: "Here again there is a city depopulated by an epidemic. We know because at the borders of the image we identify two silhouettes with a bird's beak, which represent the doctors of the plague", while the people in the city have been like sucked upwards, ballooning the figure of the Leviathan state monster, very confident of the fear he inspires.[67]

Boucheron's conclusion is that the state is always capable of obtaining an absolutely unprecedented resignation and obedience from the population: "What's complicated is that even if what everything we say about the society of surveillance is scary and true, the state obtains this obedience in the name of its most undisputed function, which is to protect the population from creeping death. That's what plenty of serious studies define as 'biolegitimacy'".

And I would add, today, a biolegitimacy boosted by widespread voluntary servitude.

THE AGE OF HAPHOPHOBIA

Michel Foucault was arguably the premier modern cartographer of the Panopticon-derived surveillance society.

---

[66] http://www.travelingintuscany.com/art/ambrogiolorenzetti/goodandbadovernment.htm

[67] https://www.college.columbia.edu/core/content/frontispiece-thomas-hobbes'-leviathan-abraham-bosse-creative-input-thomas-hobbes-1651

Then there's Gilles Deleuze. In 1978, Foucault famously declared that, "perhaps, one day, this century will be called the Deleuzian century".

Well, Deleuze is actually more 21st century than 20th. He went further than anyone else studying societies of control—where control does not come from the center or from the top but flows through micro-vigilance, even activating the desire on everyone to be disciplined and monitored: once again, voluntary servitude.

Judith Butler, talking about South Africa-based critical theorist Achille Mbembe's extraordinary *Necropolitics,* noted how he "continues where Foucault left off, tracking the lethal afterlife of sovereign power as it subjects whole populations to what Fanon called 'the zone of non-being.'" [68]

So a great deal of the intellectual debate ahead of us, borrowing from Fanon, Foucault, Deleuze, Mbembe and others, will necessarily have to focus on biopolitics and the widespread state of exception—which, as Giorgio Agamben has demonstrated, referring to Planet Lockdown, is now completely normalized.

We cannot even begin to imagine the consequences of the anthropological rupture caused by COVID-19. Sociologists for their part are already discussing how "social distancing" is an abstraction, defined and lived in quite unequal terms, and the reasons why the powers that be chose a martial vocabulary instead of forms of mobilization guided by a collective project.

And that will lead us to deeper studies of the Age of Haphophobia: our current condition of widespread fear of physical contact. Historians will be trying to analyze it in conjunction with how social phobias have evolved across centuries.

There's no question that Foucault's exhaustive mapping should be understood as a historical analysis of different techniques used by the powers that be to manage the life and death

---

[68] https://www.amazon.com/Necropolitics-Theory-Forms-Achille-Mbembe-ebook/dp/B07ZRDPSFF/ref=sr_1_1?crid=ORX7F-YPU1MVW&dchild=1&keywords=necropolitics+achille+-mbembe&qid=1587104903&sprefix=Necropolitics%2Caps%2C464&sr=8-1

of populations.[69] Between the crucial years 1975 and 1976, when he published *Discipline and Punish* (featured in this essay's epigraph) and the first volume of *History of Sexuality*, Foucault, based on the notion of "biopolitics", described the transition from a "sovereign society" to a "disciplinary society".

His main conclusion is that techniques of biopolitical government spread out way beyond the legal and punitive spheres, and now are all over the spectrum, even lodged inside our individual bodies.

COVID-19 is presenting us with a huge biopolitical paradox. When the powers that be act like they are protecting us from a dangerous disease, they are imprinting their own immunity-based definition of the community. At the same time they have the power to decide to sacrifice part of the community (elderly people left to die; victims of the economic crisis) to the benefit of their own idea of sovereignty.

The state of exception to which many parts of the world are subjected now represents the normalization of this unbearable paradox.

Living Under House Arrest

So how would Foucault see COVID-19? He would say that this epidemic radicalizes biopolitical techniques applied to a national territory, and inscribes them in a political anatomy applied to each individual body. That's how an epidemic extends to the whole population political measures of "immunization" that previously only applied—violently—to those that were considered "aliens", inside and outside the national, sovereign territory.

It's irrelevant whether SARS-Covid-2 is organic; a bioweapon; or, CIA conspiracy theory-style, part of a world domination plan. What's happening in real life is that the virus reproduces, materializes, extends and intensifies—for hundreds of millions of people—dominant forms of biopolitical and necropolitical management that were already in place. The virus is our mirror.

---

[69] https://www.mediapart.fr/journal/culture-idees/110420/les-lecons-du-virus

We are what the epidemic says we are, and how we decide to face it.

And under such extreme turbulence, as noted by philosopher Paul Preciado, we end up reaching a new necropolitical frontier—especially in the West.

The new territory of the border politics the West has been testing for years now over "The Other"—blacks, Muslims, the poor—now starts at home. It's as if Lesbos, the key entrance island for refugees in the Eastern Mediterranean coming from Turkey, now starts at the entrance of each Western apartment.

With pervasive social distancing in place, the new border is each and everyone's skin. Migrants and refugees were previously considered viruses, and only merited confinement and immobilization. But now these policies apply to whole populations. Detention centers—perpetual waiting rooms that abolish human rights and citizenship—are now detention centers inside one's own home.

No wonder the liberal West has been plunged in a state of shock and awe.

Asia Times, April 2020

12. HOW TO THINK POST-PLANET LOCKDOWN

Between unaccountability of elites and total fragmentation of civil society, COVID-19 as a circuit breaker is showing how the King—systemic design—is naked.

We are being sucked into a Danse Macabre of multiple complex systems "colliding into one another", producing all kinds of mostly negative feedback loops. [70]

What we already know for sure, as Shoshana Zuboff detailed in *The Age of Surveillance Capitalism*, is that "industrial capitalism followed its own logic of shock and awe" to conquer nature. But now surveillance capitalism "has human nature in its sights".

In *The Human Planet: How We Created the Anthropocene*, analyzing the explosion in population growth, increasing energy consumption and a tsunami of information, "driven by the positive feedback loops of reinvestment and profit", Simon Lewis and Mark Maslin of University College, London suggest that our current mode of living is the "least probable" among several options: "a collapse or a switch to a new mode of living is more likely".

As dystopia and mass paranoia seem to be the law of the (bewildered) land, Michel Foucault's analyses of **biopolitics** have never been so timely, as states across the world **take over biopower**—the control of people's life and bodies.[71, 72]

David Harvey, once again, shows how **prophetic** was Marx

---

[70] https://www.strategic-culture.org/news/2020/04/27/danse-macabre-and-a-fear-of-the-abyss-we-all-fall-down/

[71] https://criticallegalthinking.com/2017/05/10/michel-foucault-biopolitics-biopower/

[72] https://www.lemonde.fr/idees/article/2020/04/20/quand-michel-foucault-decrivait-l-etatisation-du-biologique_6037195_3232.html

not only in his analyses of industrial capitalism but somehow even forecasting the mechanics of digital capitalism: [73]

"And so Marx, in an astonishing set of passages in the *Grundrisse*—pages 650 to 710 of the Penguin edition, if you are interested—talks about the way that new technologies and knowledge become embedded in the machine: they're no longer in the laborer's brain, and the laborer is pushed to one side to become an appendage of the machine, a mere machine-minder. All of the intelligence and all of the knowledge, which used to belong to the laborers, and which conferred upon them a certain monopoly power vis-à-vis capital, disappear."

Thus, adds Harvey, "the capitalist who once needed the skills of the laborer is now freed from that constraint, and the skill is embodied in the machine. The knowledge produced through science and technology flows into the machine, and the machine becomes "the soul" of capitalist dynamism."

Living in "Psycho-Deflation"

An immediate—economic—effect of the collision of complex systems is the approaching New Great Depression. Meanwhile, very few are attempting to understand Planet Lockdown in depth—and most of all, post-Planet Lockdown. Yet a few concepts already stand out. State of exception. Necropolitics. A New Brutalism. And, as we will see, The New Viral Paradigm.

So let's review some the best and the brightest at the forefront of COVID-19 thinking. An excellent road map is provided by Sopa de Wuhan ("Wuhan Soup"), an independent collection assembled in Spanish, featuring essays, among others, by Giorgio Agamben, Slavoj Zizek, Judith Butler, David Harvey, as well as South Korean Byung-Chul Han and Spaniard Paul Preciado.[75] The

---

[73] https://www.jacobinmag.com/2020/04/david-harvey-coronavirus-pandemic-capital-economy

[74] https://www.penguinrandomhouse.com/books/275597/grundrisse-by-karl-marx

[75] https://dialektika.org/wp-content/plugins/algori-pdf-viewer/dist/web/viewer.html?file=https%3A%2F%2Fdialektika.org%2F

last two, along with Agamben, were referenced in previous essays in this running series, on the Stoics, Heraclitus, Confucius, Buddha and Lao Tzu, and contemporary philosophy examining The City under The Plague.[76],[77],[78],[79]

Franco Berardi, a 1968 student icon and professor of philosophy in Bologna, offers the concept of "psycho-deflation" to explain our current predicament. We are living a "psychic epidemic (...) generated by a virus as the Earth has reached a stage of extreme irritation, and society's collective body suffers for quite a while a state of intolerable stress: the illness manifests itself at this stage, devastating in the social and psychic spheres, as a self-defense reaction of the planetary body".

Thus, as Berardi argues, a "semiotic virus in the psycho-sphere blocks the abstract functioning of the economy, subtracting bodies from it." Only a virus would be able to stop accumulation of capital dead in its tracks: "Capitalism is axiomatic, works on a non-verified premise (the necessity of unlimited growth which makes possible capital accumulation). Every logical and economic concatenation is coherent with this axiom, and nothing can be tried outside of this axiom. There is no political way out of axiomatic Capital, there's no possibility of destroying the system", because even language is a hostage of this axiom, and does not allow the possibility of anything "efficiently extra-systemic."

So what's left? "The only way out is death, as we learned from Baudrillard". The late, great grandmaster of simulacrum was already forecasting a systemic stall back in the post-modernist 1980s.

Croatian philosopher Srecko Horvat, in contrast, offers a less conceptual and more realist hypothesis about the immediate future: "The fear of a pandemic is more dangerous than the virus

---

wp-content%2Fuploads%2F2020%2F04%2FSopa-de-Wuhan-ASPO.pdf
[76] https://asiatimes.com/2020/03/we-are-all-stoics-now/
[77] https://asiatimes.com/2020/04/it-is-disease-that-makes-health-sweet-and-good/
[78] https://asiatimes.com/2020/04/confucius-is-winning-the-covid-19-war/
[79] https://asiatimes.com/2020/04/the-city-in-a-time-of-plague/

itself. The apocalyptic images of the mass media hide a deep nexus between the extreme right and the capitalist economy. Like a virus that needs a living cell to reproduce itself, capitalism will adapt itself to the new 21st century biopolitics."[80]

For the Catalan chemist and philosopher Santiago Lopez Petit, coronavirus can be seen as a declaration of war: "Neoliberalism unabashedly dresses up as a war state. Capital is scared", even as "uncertainty and insecurity invalidate the necessity of the same state." Yet there may be creative possibilities when "obscure and paroxistic life, incalculable in its ambivalence, escapes algorithm".

OUR NORMALIZED EXCEPTION

Giorgio Agamben caused immense controversy in Italy and across Europe when he published a column in late February on "the invention of an epidemic".[81] He later had to explain what he meant.[82] But his main insight remains valid: the state of exception has been completely normalized.

And it gets worse: "A new despotism, which in terms of pervasive controls and cessation of every political activity, will be worse that the totalitarianisms we have known so far."[83]

Agamben redoubles his analyses of science as the religion of our time: "The analogy with religion is taken literally; theologians declared that they could not clearly define what is God, but in his name they dictated rules of conduct to men and did not hesitate to burn heretics. Virologists admit they don't know exactly what is a virus, but in its name they pretend to decide how human beings shall live."

Cameroonian philosopher and historian Achille Mbembe, author of two indispensable books, *Necropolitics* and *Brutalisme*,

---

[80] https://www.theguardian.com/books/2019/apr/21/srecko-horvat-poems-from-the-future-interview
[81] https://www.quodlibet.it/giorgio-agamben-l-invenzione-di-un-epidemia
[82] https://www.versobooks.com/blogs/4636-states-of-emergency-metaphors-of-virus-and-covid-19
[83] https://www.quodlibet.it/giorgio-agamben-nuove-riflessioni"

has identified the paradox of our time: "The abyss between the increasing globalization of problems of human existence and the retreat of states inside their own, old-fashioned borders."[84]

Mbembe delves into the end of a certain world, "dominated by giant calculation devices", a "mobile world in the most polymorphous, viral and near cinematic sense", referring to the ubiquity of screens (Baudrillard again, already in the 1980s) and the lexicography "which reveals not only a change of language but the end of the word."

Here we have Mbembe dialoguing with Berardi—but Mbembe takes it much further: "This end of the word, this definitive triumph of the gesture and artificial organs over the word, the fact that the history of the word ends under our eyes, that for me is the historical development par excellence, the one that COVID-19 unveils."

The political consequences are, inevitably, dire: "Part of the power politics of great nations does not lie in the dream of an automated organization of the world thanks to the manufacturing of a New Man that would be the product of physiological assemblage, a synthetic and electronic assemblage and a biological assemblage? Let's call it techno-libertarianism."

This is not exclusive to the West: "China is also on it, vertiginously."

This new paradigm of a plethora of automated systems and algorithmic decisions, "where history and the word don't exist anymore is in frontal shock with the reality of bodies in flesh and bones, microbes, bacteria and liquids of all sorts, blood included."

The West, argues Mbembe, chose a long time ago to "imprint a Dionysiac course to its history and take the rest of the world with it, even if it doesn't understand it. The West does not know anymore the difference between beginning and ending. China is also on it. The world has been plunged into a vast process of dilaceration where no one can predict the consequences."

Mbembe is terrified by the proliferation of "live manifestations

---

[84] https://www.mediapart.fr/journal/international/190420/achille-mbembe-le-monde-est-entraine-dans-un-vaste-processus-de-dilaceration

of the bestial and viral part of humanity", including racism and tribalism.

This, he adds, conforms our New Viral Paradigm.

His analysis certainly dovetails with Agamben's: "I have a feeling that brutalism is going to intensify under the techno-libertarianism drive, be it under China or hidden under the accoutrements of liberal democracy. Just like 9/11 opened the way to a generalized state of exception, and its normalization, the fight against COVID-19 will be used as a pretext to move the political even more towards the domain of security."

"But this time", Mbembe adds, "it will be a security almost biological, bearing with new forms of segregation between the 'immunity bodies' and 'viral bodies'. Viralism will become the new theatre for fractioning populations, now identified as distinct species." It does feel like neo-medievalism, a digital re-enacting of the fabulous *Triumph of Death* fresco in Palermo.[85]

POETS, NOT POLITICIANS

It's useful to contrast such doom and gloom with the perspective of a geographer. Christian Grataloup, who excels in geo-history, insists on the common destiny of humanity (here he's echoing Xi Jinping and the Chinese concept of "community of shared destiny"): "There's an unprecedented feeling of identity. The world is not simply an economic and demographic spatial system, it becomes a territory. Since the Great Discoveries, what was global was shrinking, solving a lot of contradictions; now we must learn to build it up again, give it more consistence as we run the risk of letting it rot under international tensions." [86]

It's not the COVID-19 crisis that will lead to another world—but society's reaction to the crisis. There won't be a magical night—complete with performances by "international community" pop stars—when "victory" will be announced to the former Planet Lockdown. What really matters is a long, arduous

---

[85] https://www.quodlibet.it/libro/9788874628360

[86] https://www.armand-colin.com/geohistoire-de-la-mondialisation-3ed-le-temps-long-du-monde-3e-edition-9782200602949

political combat to take us to the next level. Extreme conservatives and techno-libertarians have already taken the initiative—from refusal of any taxes on the wealthy to support the victims of the New Great Depression to the debt obsession that prevents more, necessary public spending.

In this framework, I propose to go one step beyond Foucault's biopolitics. Gilles Deleuze can be the conceptualizer of a new, radical freedom. Here is a delightful British series that can be enjoyed as if it was a serious Monty Python-ish approach to Deleuze.[87]

Foucault excelled in the description of how meaning and frames of social truth change over time, constituting new realities conditioned by power and knowledge.

Deleuze, on the other hand, focused on how things change. Movement. Nothing is stable. Nothing is eternal. He conceptualized flux—in a very Heraclitean way.

New species (even the new, AI-created *Ubermensch*) evolve in relation with their environment. It's by using Deleuze that we can investigate how spaces between things create possibilities for The Shock of the New.

More than ever, we now know how everything is connected (thank you, Spinoza). The (digital) world is so complicated, connected and mysterious that this opens an infinite number of possibilities.

Already in the 1970s, Deleuze was saying the new map—the innate potentially of newness—should be called "the virtual". The more living matter gets more complex, the more it transforms this virtual into spontaneous action and unforeseen movements.

Deleuze posed a dilemma that now confronts us all in even starker terms. The choice is between "the poet, who speaks in the name of a creative power, capable of overturning all orders and representations in order to affirm difference in the state of permanent revolution which characterizes eternal return: and that of the politician, who is above all concerned to deny that which "differs", so as to conserve or prolong an established historical order, or to establish a historical order which already calls forth in

---

[87] https://www.youtube.com/watch?v=GS35vUMhww4

the world the forms of its representation".
The time calls for acting as poets instead of politicians.

The methodology may be offered by Deleuze and Guattari's formidable *A Thousand Plateaus*—significantly subtitled "capitalism and schizophrenia", where the drive is non-linear.[88] We're talking about philosophy, psychology, politics connected by ideas running at different speeds, a dizzying non-stop movement mingling lines of articulation, in different strata, directed into lines of flight, movements of deterritorialization.

The concept of "lines of flight" is essential for this new virtual landscape, because the virtual is conformed by lines of flight between differences, in a continual process of change and freedom.

All this frenzy though must have roots—as in the roots of a tree (of knowledge). And that brings us to Deleuze's central metaphor; the rhizome, which is not just a root, but a mass of roots springing up in new directions.

Deleuze showed how the rhizome connects assemblies of linguistic codes, power relations, the arts—and crucially, biology. The hyperlink is a rhizome. It used to represent a symbol of the delightful absence of order in the internet, until it became debased as Google started imposing its algorithms. Links, by definition, always should lead us to unexpected destinations.

Rhizomes are the antitheses of those Western liberal "democracy" standard traits—the Parliament and the Senate. By contrast, trails—as in the Ho Chi Minh trail—are rhizomes. There's no masterplan. Multiple entryways and multiple possibilities. No beginning and no end. As Deleuze described it, "the rhizome operates by variation, expansion, conquest, capture, offshoot."

This can work out as the blueprint for a new form of political engagement –as the systemic design collapses. It does embody a methodology, an ideology, an epistemology and it's also a metaphor. The rhizome is inherently progressive, while traditions are static. As a metaphor, the rhizome can replace our conception of history as linear and singular, offering different histories

---

[88] https://libcom.org/files/A%20Thousand%20Plateaus.pdf"

moving at different speeds. TINA (" there is no alternative") is dead: there are multiple alternatives.

And that brings us back to David Harvey inspired by Marx. In order to embark onto a new, emancipatory path, we first have to emancipate ourselves to see that a New Imaginary is possible, alongside a new complex systems reality.

So let's chill—and deterritorialize. If we learn how to do it, the advent of the New Techno Man in voluntary servitude, remote-controlled by an all-powerful, all-seeing security state, won't be a given.

Asia Times, April 2020

Notes

Deleuze: a great writer is always like a foreigner in the language that he expresses himself, even if it's his native tongue. He does not mix another language with his own language; he carves out a non-pre-existent foreign language within his own language. He makes the language itself scream, stammer, murmur. A thought should shoot off rhizomatically—in many directions.

I have a cold. The virus is a rhizome.

Remember when Trump said this was a "foreign virus"?

All viruses are foreign—by definition.

But Trump, of course, never read *Naked Lunch* Grandmaster William Burroughs.

Burroughs: "The word is a virus."

13. THE DEEPER ROOTS OF CHINESE DEMONIZATION

Fasten your seat belts: the US Hybrid War against China is bound to go on frenetic overdrive, as economic reports are already identifying COVID-19 as the tipping point when the Asian— actually Eurasian—century truly began. [89], [90]

The US strategy remains, essentially, Full Spectrum Dominance—with the National Security Strategy obsessed by the three top "threats" of China, Russia and Iran. China, in contrast, proposes a "community of shared destiny" for mankind, mostly addressing the Global South.[91]

The predominant US narrative in the ongoing information war is now set in stone. COVID-19 was the result of a leak from a Chinese biowarfare lab. China is responsible. China lied. And China has to pay.

The new normal of non-stop China demonization is not only a tactic deployed by crude functionaries of the industrial-military-surveillance-media complex. We need to dig much deeper to discover how these attitudes are deeply embedded in Western thinking—and later migrated to the "end of History" United States. (Here are sections of an excellent study, *Unfabling the East: The Enlightenment's Encounter with Asia*, by Jurgen Osterhammel). [92]

---

[89] https://asiatimes.com/2020/03/china-locked-in-hybrid-war-with-us/
[90] https://www.mckinsey.com/featured-insights/asia-pacific/could-the-next-normal-emerge-from-asia
[91]
http://europe.chinadaily.com.cn/a/201806/23/WS5b2daa3aa310334914 1de5ea.html
[92]
https://books.google.co.th/books?id=FcmXDwAAQBAJ&pg=PA675&l pg=PA675&dq=Hegel+Interasien&source=bl&ots=BI7GSb6rjg&sig=A CfU3U3y0Ar-

Only Whites are "Civilized"

Way beyond the Renaissance, in the 17th and 18th centuries, whenever Europe referred to Asia it was essentially about religion conditioning trade. Christianity reigned supreme, so it was impossible to think by excluding God.

At the same time the absence of a transcendent religion in the Sinified world coexisting with a very well organized society deeply disturbed the Doctors of the Church—even more than those "savages" discovered in the Americas.

As it started to explore what was regarded as the "Far East", Europe was mired in religious wars. But at the same time it was forced to confront another explanation of the world—and that fed some subversive anti-religious tendencies across the Enlightenment sphere.

It was at this stage that learned Europeans started questioning Chinese philosophy—which inevitably they had to degrade to the status of a mere worldly "wisdom" because it escaped the canons of Greek and Augustinian thought. This attitude, by the way, still reigns today.

So we had what in France was described as *chinoiseries*—a sort of ambiguous admiration, where China was regarded as the supreme example of a pagan society.

But then the Church started to lose patience with the Jesuits' fascination with China. The Sorbonne was punished. A papal bull, in 1725, outlawed Christians who were practicing Chinese rites. It's quite interesting to note that Sinophile philosophers and Jesuits condemned by the Pope insisted that the "real faith" (Christianity) was "prefigured" in ancient Chinese texts—specifically Confucianism.

The European vision of Asia and the "Far East" was mostly conceptualized by a mighty German triad: Kant, Herder and Schlegel. Kant, incidentally, was also a geographer, and Herder a historian and geographer. We can say that the triad was the precursor of modern Western Orientalism. It's easy to imagine a

MC6zl69XTLGX_DVyde_CYw&hl=en&sa=X&ved=2ahUKEwje8uPSj
ZLpAhVx7XMBHVyHCEMQ6AEwAXoECAoQAQ

Borges short story featuring these three.

As much as they may have been aware of China, India and Japan, for Kant and Herder God was above all. He had planned the development of the world in all its details. And that brings us to the tricky issue of race.

Breaking away from the monopoly of religion, references to race represented a real epistemological turnaround in relation to previous thinkers. Leibniz and Voltaire, for instance, were Sinophiles. Montesquieu and Diderot were Sinophobes. None of them explained cultural differences by race. Montesquieu developed a theory based on climate. But that did not have a racial connotation—it was more like an ethnic approach.

The big break came via French philosopher and traveler Francois Bernier (1620-1688), who spent 13 years traveling in Asia and in 1671 published a book called *La Description des Etats du Grand Mogol, de l'Indoustan, du Royaume de Cachemire, etc.* Voltaire, hilariously, called him Bernier-Mogol—as he became a star telling his tales to the royal court. In a subsequent book, *Nouvelle Division de la Terre par les Differentes Especes ou Races d'Homme qui l'Habitent,* published in 1684, the "Mogol" distinguished up to five human races.

This was all based on the color of the skin, not on families or the climate. The Europeans were mechanically placed on top, while other races were considered "ugly". Afterwards, the division of humanity in up to five races was picked up by David Hume—always based on the color of the skin. Hume proclaimed to the Anglo-Saxon world that only Whites were civilized, and others are inferiors. This attitude is still pervasive. See, for instance, this pathetic diatribe recently published in Britain.[93]

Two Asias

The first thinker to actually come up with a theory of the yellow race was Kant, in his writings between 1775 and 1785, as argued on *The Great Encounter of China and the West, 1500-1800,* by

---

[93] https://www.telegraph.co.uk/politics/2020/04/22/coronavirus-will-china-welcome-ranks-civilised-world

David Mungello. Kant rates the "white race" as "superior", the "black race" as "inferior", the "copper race" as "feeble" and the "yellow race" as intermediary. The differences between them are due to a historical process, starting with the "white race", considered the most pure and original, the others being nothing but bastards.

Kant subdivided Asia by countries. For him, East Asia meant Tibet, China and Japan. He considered China in relatively positive terms, as a mix of white and yellow races.

Herder was definitely mellower. For him, Mesopotamia was the cradle of Western civilization, and the Garden of Eden was in Kashmir, "the world's paradise". His theory of historical evolution became a smash hit in the West: the East was a baby, Egypt was an infant, Greece was youth. Herder's East Asia consisted of Tibet, China, Cochin-China, Tonkin, Laos, Korea, Eastern Tartary and Japan—countries and regions touched by Chinese civilization.

Schlegel was like the precursor of a Californian 60s hippie. He was a Sanskrit enthusiast and a serious student of Eastern cultures. He said that "in the East we should seek the most elevated romanticism". India was the source of everything, "the whole history of the human spirit". No wonder this insight became the mantra for a whole generation of Orientalists. That was also the start of a dualist vision of Asia across the West that's still predominant today.

So by the 18th century we had fully established a vision of Asia as a land of servitude and cradle of despotism and paternalism in sharp contrast with a vision of Asia as a cradle of civilizations. Ambiguity became the new normal. Asia was respected as Mother of Civilizations—value systems included—and even Mother of the West. In parallel, Asia was demeaned, despised or ignored because it had never reached the high level of the West, despite its head start.

THOSE ORIENTAL DESPOTS

And that brings us to The Big Guy: Hegel. Hegel—hyper-well-informed, who used to read reports by ex-Jesuits sent from Beijing—does not write about the "Far East": only the East, which includes East Asia, essentially the Chinese world. Hegel does not care much about religion, as his predecessors did. He talks about the East from the point of view of the state and politics. In contrast to the myth-friendly Schlegel, Hegel sees the East is a state of nature in the process of reaching towards a beginning of history, unlike black Africa, which wallows in the mire of a bestial state.

To explain the historical bifurcation between a stagnant world and another one in motion, leading to the Western ideal, Hegel divided Asia in two.

One part was composed by China and Mongolia: a puerile world of patriarchal innocence, where contradictions do not develop, a world where the survival of great empires attest to its "insubstantial", immobile and ahistorical character.

The other part was *Vorderasien* ("Anterior Asia"), uniting the current Middle East and Central Asia, from Egypt to Persia. This is an already historical world.

These two huge regions are also subdivided. So in the end Hegel's *Asiatische Welt* ("Asian world") is divided by four: the plains of the Yellow and Blue rivers, the high plateaus, China and Mongolia; the valleys of the Ganges and the Indus; the plains of the Oxus (today the Amur-Darya) and the Jaxartes (today the Syr-Darya), the plateaus of Persia, the valleys of the Tigris and the Euphrates; and the Nile valley.

It's fascinating to see how in the *Philosophy of History* (1822-1830) Hegel ends up separating India from China as a sort of intermediary in historical evolution. So we have in the end, as Jean-Marc Moura showed in *L'Extrême Orient selon G. W. F. Hegel, Philosophie de l'Histoire et Imaginaire Exotique*, a "fragmented East, of which India is the example, and an immobile East, blocked in chimera, of which the Far East is the illustration."

To describe the relation between East and West, Hegel uses a couple of metaphors. One of them, quite famous, features the Sun: "The history of the world voyages from east to west, Europe thus absolutely being the end of history, and Asia the beginning". We all know where tawdry "end of history" spin-offs led us.

The other metaphor is Herder's: the East is "history's youth"— but with China taking a special place because of the importance of Confucianist principles systematically privileging the role of the family.

Nothing outlined above is of course neutral in terms of understanding Asia. The double metaphor—using the sun and maturity—could not but comfort the West in its narcissism, later inherited from Europe by the "exceptional" US. Implied in this vision is the inevitable superiority complex—in the case of the US even more acute because legitimized by the course of history.

Hegel thought that history must be evaluated under the framework of the development of freedom. Well, China and India being ahistorical, freedom does not exist, unless brought by an initiative coming from outside.

And that's how the famous "Oriental despotism" evoked by Montesquieu and the possible, sometimes inevitable, and always valuable Western intervention are, in tandem, totally legitimized. We should not expect this Western frame of mind to change anytime soon—if ever. Especially as China is about to be back as Number One.

Asia Times, May 2020

14. THE LESSONS XI LEARNED FROM THE MING DYNASTY

With Hybrid War 2.0 against China reaching fever pitch, the New Silk Roads, or Belt and Road Initiative will continue to be demonized, 24/7, as the proverbial evil communist plot for economic and geopolitical domination of the "free" world, boosted by a sinister disinformation campaign.

It's idle to discuss with simpletons. In the interest of an informed debate, what matters is to find the deeper roots of Beijing's strategy: in fact what the Chinese learned from their own rich history, and how they are applying these lessons as a re-emerging major power in the young 21st century.

Let's start with how East and West used to position themselves at the center of the world.

The first Chinese historic-geographic encyclopedia, the 2nd century BC *Classic of the Mountains and the Seas*, tells us the world was what was under the sun (*tienhia*). Composed of "mountains and seas" (*shanhai*), the world was laid out between "four seas" (*shihai*). There's only one thing that does not change: the center. And its name is "Middle Kingdom" (*Zhongguo*), that is, China.

Of course, the Europeans, in the 16th century, discovering that the earth was round, turned Chinese centrality upside down. But actually not that much (see, for instance, the 21st century Sinocentric map published in 2013). The principle of a huge continent surrounded by seas, the "exterior ocean", seems to have derived from Buddhist cosmology, where the world is described as a "four-petal lotus". But the Sinocentric spirit was powerful enough to discard and prevail over every cosmogony that might have contradicted it, such as the Buddhist, which placed India at the center.

Now compare it with Ancient Greece. Their center, based on reconstituted maps by Hippocrates and Herodotus, is a composite in the Aegean Sea, featuring the Delphi-Delos-Ionia triad.

The major split between East and West goes back to the Roman empire in the 3rd century. And it starts with Diocletian, who made it all about geopolitics. In 293, he installs a tetrarchy, with two Augustus and two Caesars, and four prefectures. Maximian Augustus is charged with defending the West (*Occidens*), with the "prefecture of Italy" having Milan as capital. Diocletian charges himself to defend the East (*Oriens*), with the "prefecture of Orient" having Nicomedia as capital.

Political religion is added to this new politico-military complex. Diocletian starts the Christian dioceses (*dioikesis*, in Greek, after his name), twelve in total. There is already a diocese of the Orient—basically the Levant and northern Egypt. There's no diocese of the Occident. But there is a diocese of Asia: basically the Western part of Mediterranean Turkey nowadays, heir to the ancient Roman provinces in Asia. That's quite interesting: the Orient is placed east of Asia.

The historical center, Rome, is just a symbol. There's no more center; in fact, the center is slouching towards the Orient. Nicomedia, Diocletian's capital, is quickly replaced by neighbor Byzantium under Constantine, and rechristened as Constantinople: he wants to turn it into "the new Rome".

When the Western Roman empire falls in 476, the empire of the Orient remains. Officially, it will become the Byzantine empire only in the year 732, while the Holy Roman Empire—which, as we know, was neither holy, nor Roman, nor an empire—resurrects with Charlemagne in 800. From Charlemagne onwards, the Occident regards itself as "Europe", and vice-versa: the historical center and the engine of this vast geographical space, which will eventually reach and incorporate the Americas.

THE SUPERSTAR ADMIRAL

We're still immersed in a—literally—oceanic debate among historians about the myriad reasons and the context that led everyone and his neighbor to frenetically take to the seas starting in the late 15th century—from Columbus and Vasco da Gama to Magellan.

But the West usually forgets about the true pioneer: iconic

Admiral Zheng He, original name Ma He, a eunuch and Muslim Hui from Yunnan province.

His father and grandfather had been pilgrims to Mecca. Zheng He grew up speaking Mandarin and Arabic and learning a lot about geography. When he was 13, he was placed in the house of a Ming prince, Zhu Di, member of the new dynasty that came to power in 1387.

Educated as a diplomat and warrior, Zheng He converted to Buddhism under his new name, although he always remained faithful to Islam. After all, as I saw for myself when I visited Hui communities in 1997 when branching out from the Silk Road, on my way to Labrang monastery in Xiahe, Hui Islam is a fascinating syncretism incorporating Buddhism, Tao and Confucianism.

Zhu Di brought down the Emperor in 1402 and took the name Yong Le. A year later he had already designated Zheng He as Admiral, and orders him to supervise the construction of a large fleet to explore the seas around China. Or, to be more precise, the "Occidental ocean" (*Xiyang*): that is, the Indian Ocean.

Thus from 1405 to 1433, roughly three decades, Zheng He led seven expeditions across the seas all the way to Arabia and Eastern Africa, leaving from Nanjing in the Yangtze and profiting from monsoon winds. They hit Champa, Borneo, Java, Malacca, Sumatra, Ceylan, Calicut, Hormuz, Aden, Jeddah/Mecca, Mogadiscio and the Eastern African coast south of the Equator.

These were real armadas—sometimes with over 200 ships, including the 72 main ones, carrying as many as 30,000 men and vast amounts of precious merchandise for trade: silk, porcelain, silver, cotton, leather products, iron utensils. The leading vessel of the first expedition, with Zheng He as captain, was 140 meters long, 50 meters wide and carrying over 500 men.

This was the original Maritime Silk Road—now revived in the 21st century. And it was coupled with another extension of the overland Silk Road: after all the dreaded Mongols were in retreat, there were new allies all the way to Transoxiana, the Chinese managed to strike a peace deal with the successor of Tamerlan. So the Silk Roads were booming again. The Ming court sent diplomats all over Asia—Tibet, Nepal, Bengal, even Japan.

The main objective of pioneering Chinese seafaring has always puzzled Western historians. Essentially, it was a diplomatic, commercial and military mix. It was important to have Chinese suzerainty recognized—and materialized via the payment of a tribute. But most of all this was about trade; no wonder the ships had special cabins for merchants.

The armada was designated as the Treasury Fleet—but denoting more a prestige operation than a vehicle for capturing riches. Yong Le was strong on soft power and economics—as he took control of overseas trade by imposing an imperial monopoly over all transactions. So in the end this was a clever, comprehensive application of the Chinese tributary system—in the commercial, diplomatic and cultural spheres.

Yong Le was in fact following the instructions of his predecessor Hongwu, the founder of the Ming ("Lights") dynasty. Legend rules that Hongwu ordered that one billion trees should be planted in Nanjing region to supply the building of a navy.

Then there's the transfer of the capital from Nanjing to Beijing in 1421, and the construction of the Forbidden City. That cost a lot of money. As much as the naval expeditions were expensive, their profits, of course, were useful.

Yong Le wanted to establish Chinese—and pan-Asian—stability via a true *Pax Sinica*. That was not imposed by force but rather by diplomacy, coupled with a subtle demonstration of power. The Armada was the aircraft carriers of the time, with cannons on sight—but rarely used—and practicing "freedom of navigation".

What the emperor wanted was allied local rulers, and for that he used intrigue and commerce rather than shock and awe via battles and massacres. For instance, Zheng He proclaimed Chinese suzerainty over Sumatra, Cochin and Ceylon. He privileged equitable commerce. So this was never a colonization process. On the contrary: before each expedition, as they were being designed, emissaries from countries to be visited were invited to the Ming court and treated, well, royally.

Those Plundering Europeans

Now compare it with the Portuguese and the European colonization—which would take place decades later across these same lands and these same seas. Between (a little) carrot and (a lot of) stick, the Europeans drove commerce mostly via massacres and forced conversions. Trade posts were soon turned into forts and military installations, something that Zheng He's expeditions never attempted.

In fact Zheng He left so many good memories that he was divinized under his Chinese name, San Bao, which means "Three Treasures", in many places in Southeast Asia such as Malacca and Ayutthaya in Thailand.

What can only be described as Judeo-Christian sadomasochism focused on imposing suffering as virtue and the only path to reach Paradise. Zheng He would never have considered that his sailors—and the populations he made contact with—had to pay this price.

So why did it all end, and so suddenly? Essentially Yong Le run out of money because of his grandiose imperial adventures. The Grand Canal—linking the Yellow River and the Yangtze basins—cost a fortune. Same for building the Forbidden City. The revenue from the expeditions was not enough.

And just as the Forbidden City was inaugurated, it caught fire, in May 1421. Bad omen. According to tradition, this means disharmony between Heaven and the sovereign, a development outside of the astral norm. Confucians used it to blame the eunuch councilors, very close to the merchants and the cosmopolitan elites around the emperor. On top of it, the southern borders were restless and the Mongol threat never really went away.

The new Ming emperor, Zhu Gaozhi, laid down the law: "China's territory produces all goods in abundance; so why should we buy abroad trinkets without any interest?" His successor Zhu Zanji was even more radical. Up to 1452, a series of imperial edicts prohibited foreign trade and overseas travel. Every infraction is considered piracy punished by death. Worse: studying foreign languages is banished, as well as teaching of Chinese to foreigners.

Zheng He dies in early 1433 or 1435: in true character, in the middle of the sea, north of Java, as he was returning from the seventh, and last, expedition. The documents and the charts used for the expeditions are destroyed, as well as the ships.

So the Ming ditched naval power and re-embraced old agrarian Confucianism, which privileges agriculture over trade, the earth over the seas, and the center over foreign lands.

No more naval retreat

The take away is that the formidable naval tributary system put in place by Yong Le and Zheng He was a victim of excess—too much state spending, peasant turbulence—as well as its own success. In less than a century, from the Zheng He expeditions to the Ming retreat, this turned out to be a massive game changer in history and geopolitics, prefiguring what would happen immediately afterwards in the long 16th century: the era when Europe started and eventually managed to rule the world.

One image is stark. While Zheng He's lieutenants were sailing the eastern coast of Africa all the way to the south, in 1433, the Portuguese expeditions were just starting their adventures in the Atlantic, also sailing south, little by little, along the Western coast of Africa. The mythical Cape Bojador was conquered in 1434.

While the seven Ming expeditions were crisscrossing Southeast Asia and the Indian Ocean since 1403, and for nearly three decades, only half a century later Bartolomeu Dias would conquer the Cape of Good Hope, in 1488, and Vasco da Gama would arrive in Goa in 1498.

Imagine one of those historical "what ifs": the Chinese and the Portuguese bumping into each other in Swahili land. After all, in 1417 it was the turn of Hong Bao, the Muslim eunuch who was Zheng He's lieutenant; and in 1498 it was Vasco da Gama's turn, guided by the "Lion of the Sea" Ibn Majid, his legendary Arab master navigator.

The Ming was not obsessed with gold and spices. For them, trade should be based on equitable exchange, under the framework of the tribute. As Joseph Needham conclusively proved in works such as *Science and Civilization in China*, the Europeans wanted way more Asian products than Orientals wanted European products, "and the only way to pay for them was gold".

For the Portuguese, the "discovered" lands were all potential colonization territory. And for that the few colonizers needed slaves. For the Chinese, slavery amounted to domestic chores at best. For the Europeans, it was all about the massive exploitation of a workforce in the fields and in mines, especially concerning black populations in Africa.

In Asia, in contrast to Chinese diplomacy, the Europeans went for massacre. Via torture and mutilations, Vasco da Gama and other Portuguese colonizers deployed a real war of terror against civilian populations.

This absolutely major structural difference is at the root of the world- system and the geo-historical organization of our world, as analyzed by crack geographers such as Christian Grataloup and Paul Pelletier. Asian nations did not have to manage—or to suffer—the painful repercussions of slavery.

So in the space of only a few decades the Chinese abdicate from closer relations with Southeast Asia, India and Eastern Africa. The Ming fleet is destroyed. China abandons overseas trade. And retreats unto itself—choosing agriculture.

Once again: the direct connection between the Chinese naval retreat and the European colonial expansion is capable of explaining the development process of the two "worlds"—the West and the Chinese center—since the 15th century.

At the end of the 15th century, there are no Chinese architects left capable of building large ships. Development of weaponry is also abandoned. In just a few decades, crucially, the Sinified world loses its vast technological advance over the West. It gets weaker. And later it would pay a huge price—symbolized in the Chinese unconsciousness by the "century of humiliation".

All of the above explains quite a few things. How Xi Jinping and the current leadership did their homework. Why China won't pull a Ming remix—and retreat again. Why and how the overland Silk Road and the Maritime Silk Road are being revived. How there won't be any more humiliations. And most of all, why the West—especially the American empire—absolutely refuses to admit the new course of history.

Asia Times, May 2020

15. HOW BIOSECURITY IS ENABLING DIGITAL NEO-FEUDALISM

Italian master thinker Giorgio Agamben has been on the—controversial—forefront examining what new paradigm may be emerging out of our current pandemic distress.

He recently called attention to an extraordinary book published seven years ago that already laid it all out. [94]

In *Tempetes Microbiennes*, Patrick Zylberman, a professor of History of Health in Paris, detailed the complex process through which health security, so far at the margins of political strategies, was sneaking into center stage in the early 2000s. [95] The WHO had already set the precedent in 2005, warning about "50 million deaths" around the world caused by the incoming swine flu. In the worst-case scenario projected for a pandemic, Zylberman predicted that "sanitary terror" would be used as an instrument of governance.

That worst-case scenario has been revamped as we speak.[96] The notion of a generalized obligatory confinement is not warranted by any medical justification, or leading epidemiological research, when it comes to fighting a pandemic. Still, that was enshrined as the hegemonic policy—with the inevitable corollary of countless masses plunged into unemployment. All that based on failed, delirious mathematical models of the Imperial College kind, imposed by powerful pressure groups ranging from the World Economic Forum to the Munich Security Conference.

Enter Dr. Richard Hatchett, a former member of the National

---

[94] https://www.quodlibet.it/giorgio-agamben-biosicurezza
[95] https://www.amazon.com/Temp%C3%AAtes-microbiennes-politique-sanitaire-transatlantique-ebook/dp/B00GP0KC34/ref=sr_1_1?dchild=1&keywords=Tempetes+Microbiennes&qid=1589452777&sr=8-1
[96] https://www.voltairenet.org/article209805.html

Security Council during the first Bush Jr. administration, who was already recommending obligatory confinement of the whole population way back in 2001. Hatchett now directs the Coalition for Epidemic Preparedness Innovations (CEPI), a very powerful entity coordinating global vaccine investment, and very cozy with Big Pharma. CEPI happens to be a brainchild of the WEF in conjunction with the Bill and Melinda Gates Foundation.

Crucially, Hatchett regards the fight against COVID-19 as a "war".[97]

The terminology—adopted by everyone from President Trump to President Macron—gives away the game. It harks back to—what else—the global war on terror, as solemnly announced in September 2001 by Donald "Known Unknowns" Rumsfeld himself.[98]

Rumsfeld, crucially, had been the chairman of biotech giant Gilead.[99] After 9/11, at the Pentagon, he got busy aiming to blur the distinction between civilians and the military when it came to GWOT. That's when "generalized obligatory confinement" was conceptualized, with Hatchett among the key players.

As much as this was a militarized Big Pharma spin-off concept, it had nothing to do with public health. What mattered was the militarization of American society to be adopted in response to bioterror—at the time automatically attributed to a squalid, tech-deprived al-Qaeda.

The current version of this project—we are at "war" and every civilian must stay at home—takes the form of what Alexander Dugin has defined as a medical-military dictatorship.

Hatchett is very much part of the group, alongside ubiquitous Anthony Fauci, the director of the National Institute of Allergy and Infectious Diseases (NIAID), very close to WHO, WEF and the Bill and Melinda Gates Foundation, and Robert Redfield,

---

[97] https://www.youtube.com/watch?v=dcJDpV-igjs

[98] https://www.nytimes.com/2001/09/27/opinion/a-new-kind-of-war.html

[99] https://www.gilead.com/news-and-press/press-room/press-releases/1997/1/donald-h-rumsfeld-named-chairman-of-gilead-sciences

director of the US chapter of the Centers for Disease Control and Prevention (CDC).

Further applications inbuilt in the project will include all-around digital surveillance, sold as health monitoring. Already implemented in the current narrative is the non-stop demonization of China, "guilty" of all things COVID-19-related. That is inherited from another tried and tested war game—the Red Dawn scheme.[100]

SHOW ME YOUR FRAGILITY

Agamben did square the circle: it's not that citizens across the West have the right to health safety; now they are juridically *forced* to be healthy. That, in a nutshell, is what biosecurity is all about.

So no wonder biosecurity is an ultra-efficient governance paradigm. Citizens had it administered down their throats with no political debate whatsoever. And the enforcement, writes Agamben, kills "any political activity and any social relation as the maximum example of civic participation."

What we are already experiencing is *social distancing as a political model*—with a digital matrix replacing human interaction, which by definition from now on will be regarded as fundamentally suspicious and politically "contagious".

Agamben has to be appalled by this "concept for the destiny of human society that in many aspects seems to have borrowed from religions in decline the apocalyptic idea of the end of the world". Economics had already replaced politics—as in everything subjected to the diktats of financial capitalism. Now the economy is being absorbed by "the new biosecurity paradigm to which every other imperative must be sacrificed."

How to fight against it? Conceptual weaponry is available, such as the courses on biopolitics taught by Michel Foucault at the College de France between 1972 and 1984. They may now be consulted via a decentralized platform set up by a collective which delightfully describes itself as "the crayfish", who "advance

---

[100] https://www.nytimes.com/2020/04/11/us/politics/coronavirus-red-dawn-emails-trump.html

laterally": a concept that does justice to great rhizomatic master Gilles Deleuze. [101], [102]

Nassim Taleb's concept of *Antifragile* is also quite helpful.[103] As he explains, "Antifragile is the antidote to Black Swans." Well, COVID-19 was a Black Swan of sorts: after all deciding elites knew something like it was inevitably coming—even as lowly Western politicians, especially, were caught totally unprepared.

Antifragile contends that because of fear (very much in evidence now) or a "thirst for order" (natural to any political power) "some human systems, by disrupting the invisible or not so visible logic of things, tend to be exposed to harm from Black Swans and almost never get any benefit. You get pseudo-order when you seek order; you only get a measure of order and control when you embrace randomness."

The conclusion is that "in the black swan world, optimization isn't possible. The best you can achieve is a reduction in fragility and greater robustness."

There's no evidence, so far, that a "reduction in fragility" in the current world-system will necessarily lead towards "greater robustness." The system has never proved to be so fragile. What we do have is plenty of indications that the system collapse is being refitted, at breakneck speed, as digital neo-feudalism.

LOST IN A BIOPOLITICAL QUARANTINE

Byung-Chul Han, the South Korean philosopher who teaches in Berlin, has attempted to lay it all out.[104] The problem is he's too much of a hostage of an idealized vision of Western liberalism.

Byung-Chul Han is correct when he notes that Asia fought COVID-19 with rigor and discipline inconceivable in the West—something that I have followed closely. But then he evokes the

---

[101] https://freefoucault.eth.link/?fbclid=IwAR2JoXgCv6k6YgQ0b6hZ4-LywnQyYCqbyfHbHS_6OtJA4W8SjO7-I3LeYKY

[102] http://thesaker.is/how-to-think-post-planet-lockdown/

[103] https://fs.blog/2014/04/antifragile-a-definition/

[104] https://blogs.mediapart.fr/jean-marc-adolphe/blog/100520/vers-un-feodalisme-digital-par-byung-chul-han

Chinese social credit system to mount an attack on China's society of digital discipline. The system unquestionably allows for biopolitical surveillance. But it's all about nuance.

The social credit system is like the formula "socialism with Chinese characteristics"; a hybrid that is effective only when responding to China's complex specificities.

The maze of facial recognition surveillance cameras; the absence of restriction to data exchanged between internet providers and the central power; the QR code that tells whether you're "red" or "green" in terms of infection; all these instruments were applied—successfully—in China to the benefit of public health.

Byung-Chul Han is forced to admit that does not take place only in China; South Korea—a Western-style democracy—is even considering that people in quarantine should wear a digital bracelet. If we talk about the different Asian models used to fight COVID-19, nuance is the norm.

The Asian-wide collectivist spirit and discipline—especially in Confucianist-influenced societies—works irrespective of the political system. At least Byung-Chul Han admits, "all these Asian particularities are systemic advantages to contain the epidemic."

The point is not that Asian disciplinary society should be seen as a model for the West. We already live in a digital global Panopticon (where's Foucault when we need him?) Social network vigilance—and censorship—deployed by the Silicon Valley behemoths has already been internalized. All our data as citizens is trafficked and instantly marketized for private profit. So yes; digital neo-feudalism was already in effect even before COVID-19.

Call it surveillance turbo-neoliberalism. Where there's no inbuilt "freedom", and it's all accomplished by voluntary servitude.

Biopolitical surveillance is just a further layer, the last frontier, because now, as Foucault taught us, this paradigm controls our own bodies. "Liberalism" has been reduced to road kill a long time ago. The point is not that China may be the model for the West.

The point is we may have been set up for an endless biopolitical quarantine without even noticing it.

Strategic Culture, May 2020

16. OUR GRIM FUTURE: RESTORED NEOLIBERALISM OR HYBRID NEOFASCISM?

With the specter of a New Great Depression hovering over most of the planet, realpolitik perspectives for a radical change of the political economy framework we live in are not exactly encouraging.

Western ruling elites will be deploying myriad tactics to perpetuate the passivity of populations barely emerging from de facto house arrest, including a massive disciplinary—in a Foucault sense—drive by states and business/finance circles.

In his latest book, *La Desaparicion de los Rituales*, Byung-Chul Han shows how total communication, especially in a time of pandemic, now coincides with total vigilance: "Domination impersonates freedom. Big Data generates a domineering knowledge that allows the possibility of intervening in the human psyche, and manipulating it. Considering it this way, the data-ist imperative of transparency is not a continuation of the Enlightenment, but its ending."[105]

This revamping of Foucault's *Discipline and Punish* coincides with reports about the demise of the neoliberal era being vastly overstated. Instead of a simplistic plunge into populist nationalism, what is on the horizon points mostly to a Neoliberalism Restoration—massively spun as a novelty, and incorporating some Keynesian elements: after all, in the post-Lockdown era, to "save" the markets and private initiative the state must not only intervene but also facilitate a possible ecological

---

[105] https://www.amazon.com/desaparici%C3%B3n-los-rituales-topolog%C3%ADa-Pensamiento-ebook/dp/B088P1V7JP/ref=sr_1_1?crid=29B25OSNXX0KN&dchild=1&keywords=la+desaparicion+de+los+rituales+herder&qid=1590671089&sprefix=La+Desaparicion+de+los+%2Caps%2C380&sr=8-1

transition.[106]

The bottom line: we may be facing a mere cosmetic approach, in which the deep structural crisis of zombie capitalism—barely moving under unpopular "reforms" and infinite debt—still is not addressed.

Meanwhile, what is going to happen to assorted fascisms? Eric Hobsbawm showed us in Age of Extremes how the key to the fascist right was always mass mobilization: "Fascists were the revolutionaries of the counter-revolution".[107]

We may be heading further than mere, crude neofascism. Call it Hybrid Neofascism. Their political stars bow to global market imperatives while switching political competition to the cultural arena.

That's what true "illiberalism" is all about: the mix between neoliberalism—unrestricted capital mobility, Central Bank diktats—and political authoritarianism. Here's where we find Trump, Modi and Bolsonaro.

FROM ANTHROPOCENE TO CAPITALOCENE

To counterpunch zombie neoliberalism, those believing another world is possible dream of a social-democratic revival; wealth redistribution; or at least neoliberalism with a human face.

That's where eco-socialism jumps in: a radical rupture with the diktats of the Goddess of the Market, the product of a healthy rebellion against ultra-authoritarian neoliberalism and illiberalism.

In sum, that could be seen as a soft adaptation of Thomas Piketty's analyses: to break the domination of capital by economic democracy, in the spirit of mid-19th century social democracy.

It's quite interesting, in this aspect, to consider *Fully*

---

[106] https://blog.mondediplo.net/quatre-hypotheses-sur-la-situation-economique

[107] https://www.amazon.com/Age-Extremes-Twentieth-Century-1914-1991/dp/0349106711/ref=sr_1_2?crid=1WEYGDAHPBS5I&dchild=1&keywords=age+of+extremes+hobsbawm&qid=1590671184&sprefix=Age+of+Extremes+%2Caps%2C396&sr=8-2

Automated Luxury Communism, by Aaron Bastani, a refreshing utopian manifesto where we see that once society is stripped off everything superfluous linked to alienation, it's still possible for everyone to find all the necessary technical means to live "in luxury" without recourse to infinity growth imposed by Capital.[108]

And that brings us to the direct link between the Anthropocene and what has been conceptualized by French economist Benjamin Coriat as the Capitalocene.[109], [110]

Capitalocene means that our current state of appalling planetary degradation should not be linked to an undefined "humanity" but "to a very defined humanity organized by a predatory economic system."

The state of the planet under the Anthropocene must be imperatively linked to the hegemonic economic system of the past two centuries: the way we developed our system of production and legitimized indiscriminate predatory practices.

The bottom line: to go beyond it, the economy must be reoriented and rebuilt, part of a "big bang in public and economic policies."

In the Anthropocene, Promethean humanity must be contained so the rape of Mother Earth can be properly tackled.

Capitalocene for its part describes Capital as the crucial root and conditioner of the current world-system. The result of the struggle against the ravaging effects of Capital will determine the

---

[108] https://www.amazon.com/Fully-Automated-Luxury-Communism-Bastani-ebook/dp/B075WCGJDW/ref=sr_1_1?dchild=1&keywords=Fully+Automated+Luxury+Communism&qid=1590671410&sr=8-1

[109] https://www.amazon.com/Human-Planet-How-Created-Anthropocene-ebook/dp/B07KMJZF42/ref=sr_1_2?crid=1BHPY0PWNHPUR&dchild=1&keywords=the+human+planet+how+we+created+the+anthropocene&qid=1590671597&sprefix=The+Human+Planet+Anthropocene%2Caps%2C398&sr=8-2

[110] https://www.mediapart.fr/journal/economie/160520/benjamin-coriat-l-age-de-l-anthropocene-c-est-celui-du-retour-aux-biens-communs?page_article=1

possible future of eco-socialism.

And that refocuses the importance of the *commons*—way beyond the opposition between private property and public property.

Coriat has shown how COVID-19 laid bare the necessity of the commons and the incapacity of neoliberalism to address it.

But how to build eco-socialism? Should it start as eco-socialism in one country (somewhere in Scandinavia)? How to coordinate it across Europe? How to fight ossified EU structures from the inside?

After all both Restored Neoliberalism and illiberalism already count on powerful states and networks. A good example is Hungary and Poland continuing to function as cogs of the German industrial supply chain.

How to prevent someone like Bill Gates to take control of a UN organization, the WHO, thus forcing it to invest in programs that fit his own personal agenda?

How to change the WTO's free market rules, according to which buying palm oil and transgenic soya contributes to the de facto deforestation of large tracts of Africa, Asia and South America? This is a state of affairs that allows wealthy nations to actually buy the destruction of ecosystems.

REVOLUTION, NOT REFORM

Even if neoliberalism was dead, and it's not, the world is still encumbered with its corpse—to paraphrase Nietzsche *à propos* of God.

And even as a triple catastrophe—sanitary, social and climatic—is now unequivocal, the ruling matrix—starring the Masters of the Universe managing the financial casino—won't stop resisting any drive towards change.

Diversionist tactics supporting an "ecological transition" fool no one.

Financial capitalism is an expert in adapting to—and profiting from—the serial crises it provokes or unleashes.

To update May 1968, what's needed is *L'Imagination au Pouvoir*. Yet it's idle to expect imagination from mere puppets such as Trump, Merkel, Macron or BoJo.

Realpolitik once again points to a post-Lockdown turbo-capitalist framework, where the illiberalism of the 1%—with fascistic elements—and naked turbo-financialization are boosted by reinforced exploitation of an exhausted and now largely unemployed workforce.

Post-Lockdown turbo-capitalism is once again reasserting itself after four decades of Thatcherization, or—to be polite—hardcore neoliberalism. Progressive forces still don't have the ammunition to revert the logic of extremely high profits for the ruling classes—EU governance included—and for large global corporations as well.

Economist and philosopher Frederic Lordon, a researcher at the French Centre national de la recherche scientifique (CNRS), cuts to the inevitable chase: the only solution would be a revolutionary insurrection.[111] And he knows exactly how the financial markets-corporate media combo would never allow it. Big Capital is capable of co-opting and sabotaging anything.

So this is our choice: it's either Neoliberal Restoration or a revolutionary rupture. And nothing in between. It takes someone of Marx's caliber to build a full-fledged, 21st century eco-socialist ideology, and capable of long-term, sustained mobilization. *Aux armes, citoyens.*

Strategic Culture, May 2020

---

[111]

https://www.youtube.com/watch?time_continue=118&v=L7HLeX16j2k&feature=emb_logo

17. BARBARISM BEGINS AT HOME

Greece invented the concept of *barbaros*. Imperial Rome inherited it as *barbarus*.

The original meaning of barbaros is rooted in language: an onomatopoeia meaning "unintelligible speech" as people go "bar bar bar" when they talk.

Homer does not refer to barbaros, but to *barbarophonos* ("of unintelligible speech"), as in those who don't speak Greek or speak very badly. Comic poet Aristophanes suggested that Gorgias was a barbarian because he spoke a strong Sicilian dialect.

Barbaru meant "foreigner" in Babylonian-Sumerian. Those of us who studied Latin in school remember *balbutio* ("stammer", "stutter", babble").

So it was speech that defined the barbarian compared to the Greek. Thucydides thought that Homer did not use "barbarians" because in his time Greeks "hadn't yet been divided off so as to have a single common name by way of contrast". The point is clear: as Stephen Kershaw delightfully demonstrated in *Barbarians: Rebellion & Resistance To The Roman Empire*, drawing from a wealth of sources ancient and modern, the barbarian was defined as in opposition to the Greek.

The Greeks invented the barbarian concept after the Persian invasions by Darius I and Xerxes I in 490 and 480-479 BC. After all they had to clearly separate themselves from the non-Greek. Aeschylus staged *The Persians* in 472 BC. That was the turning point; after that "barbarian" was everyone who was not Greek—Persians, Phoenicians, Phrygians, Thracians.

Adding to the schism, all these barbarians were monarchists. Athens, a new democracy, considered that to be the equivalent of slavery. Athens extolled "freedom"—which ideally developed reason, self-control, courage, generosity. In contrast, barbarians—and slaves—were childish, effeminate, irrational, undisciplined, cruel, cowardly, selfish, greedy, luxurious, pusillanimous.

From all of the above two conclusions are inevitable.
1. Barbarism and slavery was a natural match.
2. Greeks thought it was morally uplifting to help friends and repel enemies, and in the latter case Greeks had to enslave them. So Greeks should by definition rule barbarians.

History has shown that this worldview not only migrated to Rome but afterwards, via Christianity post-Constantine, to the "superior" West, and finally to the West's supposed "end of history": imperial America.

Rome, as usual, was pragmatic: "barbarian" was adapted to qualify anything and anyone that was not Roman. How not to relish the historical irony: for the Greeks, the Romans were also—technically—barbarians.

Rome focused more on behavior than race. If you were truly civilized, you would not be mired in the "savagery" of Nature or found dwelling in the outskirts of the world (like Vandals, Visigoths, etc.) You would live right in the center of the matrix.

So everyone who lived outside of Rome's power—and crucially, who resisted Rome's power—was a barbarian. A collection of traits would establish the difference: race, tribe, language, culture, religion, law, psychology, moral values, clothing, skin color, patterns of behavior.

People who lived in Barbaria could not possibly become civilized.

Starting from the 16th century, that was the whole logic behind the European expansion and/or rape of the Americas, Africa and Asia, the core of the *mission civilisatrice* carried as a white man's burden.

With all that in mind, a number of questions remain unanswered. Are all barbarians irredeemably barbarous—wild, uncivilized, violent? The "civilized", in many cases, may also be considered barbarian? Is it possible to configure a pan-barbarian identity? And where is Barbaria today?

The end of secularized religion

Barbarism begins at home. Alastair Crooke has shown how in an extremely polarized US "both parties" are essentially accusing each other of barbarism: "these people lie, and would stoop to any illegitimate, seditionist (i.e. unconstitutional) means, to obtain their illicit ends."[112]

Adding to the complexity, this clash of barbarisms opposes an old, conservative guard to a Woke Generation in many respects aping a Mao Cultural Revolution mindset. "Woke" could easily be interpreted as the opposite of the Enlightenment. And it's an Anglo-America phenomenon—visible among the aimless, masked, unmasked, socially disillusioned, largely unemployed and not-distanced victims of the raging New Great Depression. There is no "woke" in China, Russia, Iran or Turkey.

Yet the central Barbaria question goes way beyond street protests. The "indispensable nation" may have irretrievably lost the Western equivalent of the Chinese "mandate of heaven", dictating, unopposed, the parameters of its own construct: "universal civilization".

The fundaments of what amounts to a secularized religion are in tatters. The "narrow, sectarian pillar" of "liberal core tenets of individual autonomy, freedom, industry, free trade" was "able to be projected into a universal project—only so long as it was underpinned by *power*."

Roughly for the past two centuries this civilizational claim served as the basis for the colonization of the Global South and the West's uncontested domination over The Rest. Not anymore. Signs are creeping everywhere. The most glaring is the evolving Russia-China strategic partnership.

The "indispensable nation" lost its military cutting edge to Russia and is losing its economic/trade preeminence to China. President Putin was compelled to write a detailed essay setting the record straight on one of the pillars of the American Century: that only happened, to a large extent, due to the sacrifices of the USSR in WWII.[113]

It's quite enlightening to check how the civilizational claim is unraveling across Southwest Asia—what the Orientalist perspective defines as the Middle East.

In a paroxysm of missionary zeal, the self-appointed heir to

---

[112] https://www.strategic-culture.org/news/2020/06/24/americas-psychic-scission-defines-global-politics-too/
[113] http://en.kremlin.ru/events/president/news/63527

imperial Rome—call it Rome on the Potomac—is bent, via the Deep State, on destroying by all means necessary the allegedly "barbarian" Axis of Resistance: Tehran, Baghdad, Damascus and Hezbollah. Not by military means, but via economic apocalypse.

This testimony, by an European religious figure working with Syrians, concisely shows how the Caesar Act sanctions—perversely depicted as a "Civilian Protection Act" and drafted under Obama in 2016—are designed to harm and even starve local populations, deliberately steering them towards civil unrest. [114]

James Jeffrey, the US envoy to Syria, even rejoiced, on the record, that sanctions against "the regime" have "contributed to the collapse" of what is essentially Syrian livelihood.[115]

Rome on the Potomac sees the Axis of Resistance as Barbaria. For one hegemonic US faction, they are barbarous because they dare to reject the superior, "moral" American civilization claim. For another no less hegemonic faction, they are so outright barbarian that only regime change would redeem them. A great deal of "enlightened" Europe happens to supports this interpretation, slightly sweetened by humanitarian imperialism overtones.

THE WALL OF ALEXANDER

It's Iraq all over again. In 2003, the beacon of civilization launched Shock and Awe on "barbarian" Iraq, a criminal operation based on entirely falsified intel—very much like the recent chapter of never-ending Russiagate, where we see malign Russkies playing the role of paymasters to Taliban with the intent of killing (occupying) US soldiers.

This "intel"—corroborated by no evidence, and parroted uncritically by corporate media—comes from the same system that tortured innocent prisoners in Guantanamo until they confessed to anything; lied about WMDs in Iraq; and weaponized

---

[114] http://freesuriyah.eu/?p=4365&fbclid=IwAR0kqv8VUCjCaV4C-YsoqjSFF7aVzuDE4LUKXiHbXRn_PQASB3-00ZUXipPM
[115] https://english.aawsat.com/home/article/2324806/us-official-sanctions-contributed-devaluation-syrian-pound

and financed Salafi-jihadis—sweetened as "moderate rebels"—to kill Syrians, Iraqis and Russians.

It's no wonder that across Iraq in 2003, I never ceased to hear from Sunnis and Shi'ites alike that the American invaders were more barbarous than the Mongols in the 13th century.

One of the key targets of the Caesar Act is to close for good the Syrian-Lebanese border. An unintended consequence is that this will lead Lebanon to get closer to Russia-China. Hezbollah's secretary-general Hassan Nasrallah has already made it very clear.[116]

Nasrallah added a subtle historical insight—emphasizing how Iran has always been the strategic, cultural go-between for China and the West: after all, for centuries, the language of choice along the Ancient Silk Roads was Persian. Who's the barbarian now?

The Axis of Resistance, as well as China, know that a festering wound will have to be tackled: the thousands of Salafi-jihadi Uighurs scattered across the Syria-Turkey border, which could become a serious problem obstructing the overland, northern Levant route of the New Silk Roads.[117]

In Libya, part of the Greater Middle East, utterly destroyed by NATO and turned into a wasteland of warring militias, the "leading from behind" fight against Barbaria will take the form of perpetuating the warring—local populations be damned. The playbook is a faithful replay of the 1980-1988 Iran-Iraq war.

In a nutshell, the "universal civilization" project has been able to utterly destroy the "barbarian" state structures of Afghanistan, Iraq, Libya and Yemen. But that's where the buck stops.

Iran has drawn the new line in the sand. Profiting from the hardened experience of living four decades under US sanctions, Tehran sent a large business delegation to Damascus to schedule the supply of necessities and is "breaking the fuel siege of Syria by sending several oil tankers"—much as the breaking of the US blockade on Venezuela. The oil will be paid in Syrian lira.[118]

---

[116] https://www.voltairenet.org/article210259.html

[117] https://ejmagnier.com/2020/02/11/syria-imposes-the-astana-deal-by-force-as-turkish-russian-tensions-rise/

[118] https://ejmagnier.com/2020/06/23/the-us-soft-war-on-iran-and-its-

So Caesar Act is actually leading Russia-China-Iran—the three key nodes in myriad strategies of Eurasia integration—to get closer and closer to the "barbarian" Axis of Resistance. A special feature is the complex diplomatic-energy ties between Iran and China—also part of a long-term strategic partnership. That includes even a new railway to be built linking Tehran to Damascus and eventually Beirut (part of BRI in Southwest Asia)—which will also be used as an energy corridor.

On Surah 18 of the Holy Quran, we find the story of how Alexander the Great, on his way to the Indus, met a faraway people who "could scarcely understand any speech". Well, barbarians.

The barbarians told Alexander the Great they were being threatened by some people they called—in Arabic—Gog and Magog, and asked for his help. The Macedonian suggested they get a lot of iron, melt it down and build a giant wall, following his own design. According to the Quran, as long as Gog and Magog were kept away, behind the wall, the world would be safe.

But then, on Judgment Day, the wall would fall. And hordes of monsters would drink away all the waters of the Tigris and the Euphrates.

Buried beneath some hills in northern Iran, the fabled Sadd-i-Iskandar ("Wall of Alexander") is still there. Yes, we will never know what sort of monsters, engendered by the sleep of reason, lurk across Barbaria.

Asia Times, July 2020

---

allies-is-turned-against-washington/

18. Eurasia, The Hegemon, and The Three Sovereigns

There are essentially four truly sovereign states in the world today, at least amongst the major powers: the United States, the Russian Federation, the People's Republic of China, and the Islamic Republic of Iran.

These four sovereigns—I call them the Hegemon and the Three Sovereigns—stand at the vanguard of the ultra-postmodern world, characterized by the supremacy of data algorithms and techno-financialization ruling over politics.

It so happens that these Three Sovereigns constitute the three key nodes of Eurasian integration and the top three existential "threats" to the Hegemon, according to the US National Security Strategy.

The story of the young twenty-first century will continue to revolve around the clash between the United States—joined by its NATO subsidiary—and these three independent Eurasian powers. It is imperative therefore for the core states that make up the Silk Road region to grasp the strategic conceptual trends that stand behind the geopolitical interplay taking place in what Zbigniew Brzezinski rightly called the "world's axial supercontinent."

Against all odds, the Silk Road region has managed to become, notwithstanding the few obvious exceptions, a bastion of stability in an increasingly vacillating and unpredictable world. In the coming period, regional leaders will need to figure out how to build upon this foundation of stability to create a region defined by the sort of dynamism that reinforced the stability that serves as the basis of the entire construction. They will have to do so in the context of an ongoing data revolution that is reconceptualizing the understanding of sovereignty.

So it is with this introduction that I would ask readers to imagine this admittedly unorthodox headline: "Michel Foucault to the rescue: where shall we find the real Sovereign, now?" To unpack this mysterious phrase we will need to turn to a number of other contemporary thinkers and concepts.

The most influential philosopher currently writing in the German language—who happens to be a South Korean by birth—is Byung-Chul Han. He has recently been making the argument that the effects of the COVID-19 pandemic may very well lead to a redefinition of the concept of sovereignty (in his words: "the sovereign is the one who resorts to data").

With this in mind, let us attempt to mix this insight with what may constitute the three major interlocking issues further on down the rocky road of 21st century geopolitics: the appalling management of the COVID-19 crisis; the possible emergence of a new paradigm; and the overall reconfiguration of the international system.

A useful starting point may be to explore some of the ideas contained in *Necropolitics* (2019) by Achille Mbembe, the Sorbonne-educated Cameroonian philosopher and political theorist. The book presents the genealogy of our contemporary world, plagued by ever-increasing inequality, militarization, and enmity, as by a resurgence of retrograde forces determined to exclude and subjugate progressive attempts to build a more equitable and just system. One of the main trusts of the book is Mbembe's attempt to pierce far beyond sovereignty as interpreted in conventional political science and predominant international relations narratives.

Mbembe revisits Michel Foucault's famous lectures delivered at the College de France in 1975-1976, in which he conceptualized biopower as the domain of life over which power has absolute control.

Foucault himself defined biopower as "an explosion of numerous and diverse techniques for achieving the subjugation of bodies and the control of populations." On this basis, Mbembe develops the relation of biopower with sovereignty—*Imperium*—and the state of exception, as conceptualized by Giorgio Agamben. Mbembe tells us that, "the ultimate expression of sovereignty is the production of general norms by a body (the demos) comprising free and equal individuals." Then these individuals are considered as full subjects capable of self-understanding, self-consciousness, and self-representation.

Thus politics is defined as a project of autonomy and as the process of reaching an agreement within a collective, through communication and recognition. The problem is that in ultra-postmodernity, this whole project has been shattered. Relations have been debased to a permanent state of Hybrid War.

Late modernity revolved around a paradigm whereby reason is the truth of the subject and politics is the exercise of reason in the public sphere. And that exercise of reason corresponds to the exercise of freedom—a key element for individual autonomy.

Mbembe wistfully evokes the "romance of sovereignty" that rests on the belief that the subject is both master and controlling author of his own meaning. Exercising sovereignty is about society's capacity for self-creation with recourse to institutions inspired by specific social and imaginary significations, as Cornelius Castoriadis reminded us in *The Imaginary Institution of Society* (1975). But, in fact, sovereignty is above all defined as the right to kill in defiance of international law. This has become a characteristic of the various expeditionary adventures conducted around the world for decades by the Hegemon.

Foucault's notion of biopower must be freshly examined in the myriad declinations of the state of exception and the state of siege. Biopower in Foucault divides people into those allowed to live and those who must die. Now biopower is applied in much more subtle ways—especially through economic sanctions capable of provoking slow death.

Control presupposes a distribution of human species into groups, a subdivision of the population into subgroups, and the establishment of a biological divide between these subgroups. Foucault used to relate the whole process to racism—a concept that was not simply based on the color of one's skin, as in the black/white dichotomy, but one that took into account all sorts of racial and ethnic gradations presupposing Western hegemony.

Now, Mbembe stresses how "racial thinking more than class thinking (where class is an operator defining history as an economic struggle between classes) has been the ever-present shadow hovering over Western political thought and practice, especially when the point was to contrive the inhumanity of foreign peoples and the sort of domination to be exercised over them." For Foucault, racism is above all a technology allowing the exercise of biopower. In the economy of biopower, the function of racism is to regulate the distribution of death and to enable the state's killing machine. It goes without saying that this biopower mechanism is inbuilt in the functioning of all modern states.

Mbembe reminds us how the material premise of Nazi extermination is to be found in colonial imperialism and in the serialization of technical mechanisms for outing people to death, developed between the industrial revolution—as shown, for instance, in Priya Satia's *Empire of Guns* (2018)—and the First World War. That's how the working classes and the "stateless people" of the industrial world found their equivalent in the "savages" or "barbarians" of the colonial world.

There is no question that an adequate historical narrative of the rise of modern terror—and modern terror in slow motion—needs to address the legacy of slavery, one of the first instances of biopolitical experimentation.

As Mbembe stresses, the structure of the plantation system—and its dire consequences—express the paradoxical figure of the state of exception. The slave condition includes loss of home, loss of rights over his/her body, and loss of political status. Think of Nagorno-Karabakh ("Artsakh is Armenia, and that's it") or Palestine, for that matter ("there are no Palestinians"). Loss is equal to absolute domination, alienation and social death—as in de facto expulsion from humanity. The colony—and the apartheid system—operates a synthesis between massacre and bureaucracy, that "incarnation of Western rationality" as noted by Hannah Arendt in *The Origins of Totalitarianism* (1951).

The point is that the technologies that produced Nazism have a strong affinity to those that resulted in the plantation and the colony. And as Foucault showed, Nazism and Stalinism only amplified a series of already existing mechanisms of Western European social and political formation: subjugation of the body, health regulations, social Darwinism, eugenics, medico-legal theories on heredity, degeneration, and race.

The colony thus represents a place in which sovereignty

fundamentally consists in exercising a power outside the law and in which "peace" assumes the face of Endless War. Not by accident did the Pentagon reinvent the concept—the terminology used was "the long war"—immediately after 9/11. This ties in with the definition of sovereignty by Carl Schmitt in the early 20th century: the "power to decide the state of exception." Think of the Hegemon's hot wars (Afghanistan, Iraq, Libya) and proxy wars (Syria, Yemen).

Late modern colonial occupation is a disciplinary, biopolitical, and necropolitical mix. Mbembe concludes that the "most accomplished form of necropower" is the neo-colonial occupation of Palestine, featuring no continuity between ground and the sky; drones crammed with sensors; aerial reconnaissance jets; early warning Hawkeye procedures; assault helicopters; satellites; techniques of hologrammatization; medieval siege warfare adapted to the networked sprawl of urban refugee camps and systematic bulldozing.

Obviously, there are other necropower examples, as well. Zygmunt Bauman noted already in the 2000s that the wars of globalization are not about conquest, acquisition, and takeover of territory. Mbembe stresses they are, "ideally, hit-and-run affairs," manifestations of which have been seen recently in parts of the Silk Road region.

What is emerging alongside conventional armies—NATO in Afghanistan surrounded by a maze of contractors, for instance—are "war machines," as in a corporate bastardization of the concept elaborated in *A Thousand Plateaus* (1980) by Gilles Deleuze and Félix Guattari.

This metamorphosis defines, for instance, the mini-galaxy of "moderate rebels" in Syria. They borrow from regular armies and incorporate new elements adapted to the principle of segmentation and deterritorialization—a mix between a political organization and a mercantile enterprise, operating through capture and depredation.

Mbembe shows how necropolitics is reconfiguring the relations between resistance (think the Axis of Resistance: Iran, Iraq, Syria, Hezbollah), sacrifice (as in fighting ISIS/Daesh jihadi fanaticism), and terror (as applied by strands of "moderate rebels"). The Hegemon, for its part, continues to practice Necropower—as in deploying weapons in the interest of maximally destroying people's living conditions and creating what Mbembe defines as "death-worlds," namely unique forms of social existence in which vast populations have the status of living dead.

Byung-Chul-Han takes the conceptual consequences of Mbembe's analysis one step beyond. Necropower is the least of our problems when the whole Kantian world—predicated on a faith that humanity, as a free and autonomous subject, shapes the formative and legislative instance of knowledge—is dead.

The new emerging paradigm is the product of a Copernican anthropological turn. Data is the New Sovereign. Man has abdicated the role of producer of knowledge to the profit of data. Data-ism thus finishes off whatever lineaments of idealism and humanism had characterized the Enlightenment. Knowledge is now produced by a binary (war) machine—and that, of course, applies to Necropower as well. Man himself has been reduced to a mere and calculable accumulation of data.

The consequence is inevitable: total communication coincides with total vigilance. We have entered the realm of what may be called "Discipline and Punish 2.0." Our whole reality—or, to evoke the late Jean Baudrillard, our whole simulacra—is subjected to the logic of non-stop for-profit production taking place under relentless pressure.

Algorithms are capable of numerization yet are incapable of producing a narrative. To think is way more substantive than to merely calculate. There is an erotic aspect to thinking, which traces its roots back to classical Greek philosophy: remember "Eros, the most ancient God according to Parmenides," to quote Martin Heidegger. Deep down, to exercise free thinking is to play, as Georges Bataille used to say. "We are all players," Baudrillard stressed, "in ardent wait for those occasionally rational chains to dissipate."

To think is essentially subversive. Calculus is erotic and rectilinear; thinking implies a sinuous trajectory: *Homo ludens*. Thus Byung-Chul-Han's formulation: from Myth to Data, real, critical, creative thinking totally lost its playful element.

And so we come to the COVID-19 pandemic. Here it would be

helpful to refer to the writings of Giorgio Agamben, who did in fact square the circle: it's not that citizens across the West have the right to health safety, he has written, it's the fact that now they have been juridically forced to be healthy. And that, in a nutshell, is what biosecurity—a data process—is all about.

Obviously, there are conventional advantages to biosecurity. Nonetheless—and equally obviously—we cannot escape the fact that biosecurity is an ultra-efficient governance paradigm. Citizens have had it imposed with virtually no political debate whatsoever. The enforcement, as Agamben has noted, killed "any political activity and any social relation as the maximum example of civic participation [in the West]."

That is how the West came to experience social distancing as an entirely new, unprecedented political model—with a (flawed) digital matrix replacing human interaction, which by definition from now on will be regarded as fundamentally suspicious and politically "contagious."

Agamben had to be appalled by this "concept for the destiny of human society that in many aspects seems to have borrowed from religions in decline the apocalyptic idea of the end of the world." In ultra-postmodernity, economics had already replaced politics—as in everything subjected to the diktats of financial capitalism. Now the economy is being absorbed by "the new biosecurity paradigm to which every other imperative must be sacrificed."

Nassim Taleb's concept of "antifragile," elaborated in 2012, might be helpful here. "Antifragility is beyond resilience or robustness. The resilient resists shocks and stays the same; the antifragile gets better," he writes. "This property is behind everything that has changed with time: evolution, culture, ideas, revolutions, political systems, technological innovation, cultural and economic success, corporate survival, [...] even our own existence as a species on this planet." The classic example of something antifragile is Hydra, the Greek mythological creature that has numerous heads. When one is cut off, two grow back in its place.

As he explains, "Antifragile is the antidote to Black Swans." The modern world may increase technical knowledge, but it will also make things more fragile. "Black Swans hijack our brains, making us feel we 'sort of' or 'almost' predicted them, because they are retrospectively explainable. We don't realize the role of these Swans in life because of this illusion of predictability." The potency of randomness is underestimated: "when we see it, we fear it and overreact. Because of this fear and thirst for order, some human systems, by disrupting the invisible or not so visible logic of things, tend to be exposed to harm from Black Swans and almost never get any benefit."

The central point of the Black Swan problem, Taleb says, "is that the odds of rare events are simply not computable." Yet COVID-19 was a Black Swan, but only of a sort: after all, deciding elites knew for quite some time that something like it was inevitably coming—even as mediocre Western politicians were caught totally unprepared.

Antifragile might lead, optimistically, to a reduction in fragility and greater robustness. Yet there is no evidence, so far, that a "reduction in fragility" within the framework of the current international system, such as it is, will invariably lead towards "greater robustness." In fact, the international system has never been so fragile as it is presently. What we do have is plenty of indications that the system collapse is being refitted, at breakneck speed, as digital neo-feudalism. Once again: we are witnessing the onset of data as the New Sovereign.

Asian-wide collectivist spirit and discipline in the fight against COVID-19—especially in Confucianist-influenced societies—has worked irrespective of the political system within which the countries in question are organized. But the key point is not that Asian disciplinary society might be seen as a model for the West. We already live in a digital global Panopticon—a sort of Foucault- on-steroids situation. Social network vigilance—and censorship—deployed by the Silicon Valley behemoths has already been internalized. All our data as citizens is trafficked and instantly marketized for private profit. So digital neo-feudalism was already in effect even before the onset of COVID-19.

In previous writings I had called it "surveillance turbo-neoliberalism" in which there is no inbuilt "freedom" in the Western sense and everything is accomplished by voluntary servitude. Biopolitical surveillance is just a further layer in the whole process—the final frontier, so to speak—because now, as Foucault taught us, this paradigm controls our own bodies. "Liberalism" has been reduced to road kill a long time ago. The point is not that China may eventually become the model for the West but rather that the West may have been set up for an endless biopolitical quarantine without people even noticing it.

In realpolitik terms, the post-lockdown turbo-capitalist framework points to a calcification of the sort of illiberalism privileged by the one percent in the West, coupled with naked turbo-financialization boosted by the reinforced exploitation of an exhausted and now increasingly unemployed workforce.

Throughout the pandemic, the plutocrats at the helm of hegemonic capital interests—well-equipped to co-opt and even sabotage anything that threatens their standing—have not stood on the sides. Consider the long planned World Economic Forum's initiative, scheduled to take place in mid-2021, called The Great Reset. According to the World Economic Forum, it is defined as a "commitment to jointly and urgently build the foundations of our economic and social system for a more fair, sustainable and resilient future."

This "reset" is meant to elaborate a "new social contract centered on human dignity, social justice and where societal progress does not fall behind economic development" by "connecting key global governmental and business leaders in Davos with a global multi-stakeholder network in 400 cities around the world for a forward-oriented dialogue driven by the younger generation." So the planet may rest in peace: Davos Man will push the button, and a Brave New World will enlighten us all.

But let us come back to the real world. Apart from the Hegemon, arguably there are only three real Sovereigns left in ultra-postmodernity: Russia, China and Iran. NATO members are not more than unevenly glorified vassals, as US President Donald Trump has ironically made rather evident in various public statements.

Once again: these Three Sovereigns happen to constitute, simultaneously, the three key nodes of Eurasia integration and are defined as constituting the top three existential "threats" to the

Hegemon, according to the US National Security Strategy. The story of the young twenty-first century will continue to revolve around the clash between the Hegemon and Eurasia's three independent major powers.

At his June 2020 Moscow Parade speech celebrating the seventy-fifth anniversary of the allied victory in Second World War, Vladimir Putin, while stressing "friendship and trust between nations" and the necessity to achieve a "common reliable security system," made it clear that the Western neoliberal system is facing the worst financial meltdown in recorded history. He underscored the point that a new international system will, by necessity, have to be brought online. Otherwise, he noted, the world will be facing the imposition of a de facto hybrid neofascist "solution."

Russia, China, and Iran are not intended to become constitutive elements of the Davos "Great Reset." As it stands, Moscow and Beijing are more like playing "dragon in the fog"—a delightful Chinese concept evoked by former Kremlin adviser Alexey Chesnakov according to which a strong player, in a complex space, is able to strike at his competitors at any moment from an unexpected angle.

This is the key takeaway from the lengthy telephone conversation held between Putin and Xi Jinping in mid-July in which they discussed virtually all aspects of the evolving Russo-Chinese strategic partnership—a conversation that took place against the background of Russia's constitutional referendum and the announcement of the new national security law in Hong Kong. According to the official Chinese readout of the call, Xi referred explicitly to "external sabotage and intervention" in his discussion with Putin.

As much as "external sabotage and intervention" is bound to reach fever pitch, the Belt and Road Initiative, complete with all its various branches and derivations—polar, space, health, information—will continue to be deployed as the Chinese roadmap for the 21st century, which has seen partnerships established with virtually all the countries of the Silk Road region, as well as many, many more.

In parallel with BRI, Russia is advancing the Eurasia Economic

Union (EAEU) as well as its own New Silk Road vectors focused on Arctic development, space exploration, biospheric engineering, and fusion power. BRI and EAEU are in a process of congruence and achieving, slowly but surely, some sort of merger. For instance, the development of the Russian Far East is one of the great projects of the 21st century, which is conceived to be achieved in partnership with China, Japan, South Korea, and India.

The interpolation of BRI and EAEU is an open system, based on a set of principles, with a special place for "win-win" partnerships in trade, economics, and politics. The Western equivalent would be the Westphalian system that established modern nation-states in 1648.

The Peace of Westphalia is in fact an open system that enshrined the concept of state sovereignty into international law, and that centuries later was set in stone by the United Nations Charter. It is a "win-win" partnership in the sense that every state, whatever its size and economic importance, has an equal right to sovereignty.

So any rumblings by Western oligarchies hinting at a post-Westphalian system—something that was somewhat advanced in the past several decades by humanitarian imperialist interventions of the Kosovo and Libya kind—in fact constitute a threat to what until recently was established as a moderate, best-of-possible-worlds level playing field.

On the "external sabotage and intervention" front, China seems to be overtaking Russia as a primary focus of American (and to a much lesser extend European) opprobrium. Virtually every move seems to be converging towards provoking a fragmentation of China, with the intention of atrophying it geopolitically to a level, in the wild dreams of some Western policymakers, comparable to the "century of humiliation."

Yan Xuetong, Dean of the Institute of International Relations at Tsinghua University, recently argued that Cold War 2.0, unlike the original Cold War, will be essentially a technological competition. As a direct hot war is unthinkable, considering the inevitability of nuclear escalation, myriad forms of Hybrid War, some already in effect, will proliferate.

That, in itself, will be already crystallizing the onset of a "post-Westphalian" process, with scores of nation states dragged into a decoupling scenario and forced to take sides. Reference models will vanish. Xenophobia and hyper-nationalism with fascistic traits will prevail. International law—already thrown in the dustbin of history with the onset, ironically, of the doctrine of the end of history by the Hegemon around the time of the fall of the Berlin Wall—will be rendered meaningless.

For at least a few decades the Hegemon, based on its global military reach, was able to offer a geopolitical and geoeconomic framework in which at least some selected players enjoyed political and economic benefits. China—in terms of trade and investment—was one of them.

But since Xi's 2013 announcement establishing the vision of BRI as a matchless roadmap for globalization 2.0—in fact, as the only credible game in town—the process of decoupling became all but inevitable.

BRI is the embryo of a transformation of the international system—a soft reinvention of capitalism. What Putin had proposed at the Munich Security Conference in the 2000s (unsuccessfully, it turned out) was re-packaged and re-proposed by Xi in the 2010s. This time, what was on offer quickly found an audience in vast parts of not only the Silk Road region but also amongst the members of the Non-Aligned Movement (NAM) and other parts of the Global South (not to mention member states of the European Union), as it emphasized China's civilizational discipline and ability to independently innovate.

It is as if in a post-Planet Lockdown environment, the world may need to keep pace with China or risk getting left in the dust.

With this we may turn for a moment to Iran. The case of Iran is extremely complex—not least because of the delicate political balancing inbuilt in a unique Shia theo-democracy. Even facing the Hegemon's relentless "maximum pressure," Supreme Leader Ayatollah Ali Khamenei has managed to regiment society by drawing on the formidable Shia ethic of resistance. As a priceless geostrategic prize, and confronted not only by the Hegemon but also Israel and assorted Arab regimes, Iran has at least managed to improve relations with key neighbors (and important New Silk Road actors) Turkey and Pakistan.

Yet the game-changers are really Russia and China. The Three Sovereigns, slowly but surely, are on their way to harmonize their different payment systems; the possibility is open for these to eventually merge in the near future, bypassing the US dollar. After the end of the Iran nuclear deal-related UN sanctions this year, Iran may be admitted as a full member of the Shanghai Cooperation Organization. The recently announced 25-year strategic partnership with China, which covers multiple fields, solidifies Iran as a key New Silk Road node and enhances China's national security in the context of firmly aligning with a reliable energy provider.

What should lie ahead is an enhanced Turkey-Iran-Pakistan partnership, interlinked with the SCO agenda, advancing the integration of West Asia with South Asia in which Iran plays the double role of energy provider and key transit route. As much as investing in connectivity with the Arab world—the Iran-Iraq-Syria-Lebanon road and rail axis—Tehran should also advance the same connectivity role with Central Asia, via the Caspian Sea and also overland to Azerbaijan and Turkmenistan. All of this should be conducted in strictly pragmatic terms, which implies toning down what remains of Islamic revolutionary rhetoric.

Largely self-sufficient, even under harsh sanctions, with a well-educated young population and profiting from excellent technical knowledge, Iran is ideally positioned to revive the role it played along the Silk Road in ancient times. A political, economic, diplomatic, military, and connectivity alliance of the Three Sovereigns is the essential building block of Eurasia integration. Build it, and they will come.

Asia is now one step beyond conceptualizing and embarking on a full-on implementation of economic uplift for the whole of Eurasia, with an African extension.

As the Silk Road region, in particular, invests in its integration, the EU fragments. Germany, even if not a Sovereign but a de facto NATO vassal, may eventually assert its regional hegemony by crushing even more the illusions of the mini-sovereigns—as in the eurozone, where the minis are absolutely impotent to determine economic policies in accordance with their national interest.

In the event that Europe, crippled by north-south and east-west internal corrosion, is prevented from profiting from its status as the largest economic block in the world, it will be inexorably reduced to no more than an inconsequent Far Western Asia. Talk about Revenge of History redux.

As it stands, the mostly American playbook has featured sanctions and trade wars—especially against the Three Sovereigns. It is misguided to qualify it as the advent of a new illiberal order. Russia and China—and to a certain extent Iran—were asking for a rethink of the post-1945 (and post-1989) international system, alongside others like Turkey. They were flatly rebuked. That only served to accelerate the logical flow of history—which is the progressive integration of the "heartland," in H.J. Mackinder's formulation.

It was the Hegemon that in fact acted as an illiberal power—when we observe how trade wars and sanctions are now configured as the new normal, directed at entire populations of nations arbitrarily deemed as enemies (e.g. Iran, Syria, Venezuela, Yemen). Necropower is inbuilt in the era of Total Economic War.

A not entirely unimportant corollary to this is the fact that there is no evidence that UN Security Council reform will be allowed by the five permanent members. Yet the real gap is not between the UN nuclear club and the rest, considering the nuclear capabilities of India, Pakistan, North Korea, and Israel. The real gap is between the Three Sovereigns—Russia, China, and Iran—and a Hegemon still conditioned by the logic of perpetual war and the refusal to admit the "unipolar moment" has come and gone. In this lies the heart of Cold War 2.0.

Mbembe concisely encapsulated the drama of the young 21st century as the "extreme fragility of all. And of the All." With necropower and data-as-sovereign tightening its grip, what passes now for "democracy" in the West is being reduced to a hollowed out shell, unpredictable, paranoid, corroded by the marriage of manufactured consent and political correctness, devoid of substantive meaning and increasingly lacking in justification: a mere (and increasingly outdated) ornament. As the countries of the Silk Road region continue to invest in various integration strategies to ensure the heartland become a geopolitical player in its own right, they would be wise to keep in mind the rebalancing taking place between the Hegemon and the Three Sovereigns in the context of the construction of our ultra-postmodern world.

This is a slightly modified version of an essay originally published in the Fall 2020 edition of *Baku Dialogues*. [119]

---

[119] https://bakudialogues.ada.edu.az/articles/eurasia-the-hegemon-and-the-three-sovereigns

19. CLASH OF CIVILIZATIONS, REVISITED

Late afternoon in May 29, 1453, Sultan Mehmet, the third son of Murad, born of a slave-girl—probably Christian—in the harem, fluent in Turkish, Arabic, Greek, Latin, Persian and Hebrew, followed by his top ministers, his imams and his bodyguard of Janissaries, rides slowly towards the Great Church of St Sophia in Constantinople.

It's unlikely that Sultan Mehmet would be sparing a thought for Emperor Justinian, the last of quite a breed: a true Roman Emperor in the throne of Byzantium, a speaker of "barbarous" Greek (he was born in Macedonia) but with a Latin mind.

Much like Sultan Mehmet, Justinian was quite the geopolitician. Byzantium trade was geared towards Cathay and the Indies: silk, spices, precious stones. Yet Persia controlled all the caravan routes on the Ancient Silk Road. The sea route was also a problem; all cargo had to depart from the Persian Gulf.

So Justinian had to bypass Persia.

He came up with a two-pronged strategy: a new northern route via Crimea and the Caucasus, and a new southern route via the Red Sea, bypassing the Persian Gulf.

The first was a relative success; the second a mess. But Justinian finally got his break when a bunch of Orthodox monks offered him to bring back from Asia some precious few silkworm eggs. Soon there were factories not only in Constantinople but also in Antioch, Tyre and Beirut. The imperial silk industry—a state monopoly, of course—was up and running.

A fantastic mosaic in Ravenna from the year 546 depicts a Justinian much younger than 64, his age at the time. He was a prodigy of energy—and embellished Constantinople non-stop. The apex was the Church of St. Sophia—the largest building in the world for centuries.

So here we have Sultan Mehmet silently proceeding with his slow ride all the way to the central bronze doors of St Sophia.

He dismounts and picks up a handful of dust and in a gesture of humility, sprinkles it over his turban.

Then he enters the Great Church. He walks towards the altar.

A barely perceptible command leads his top imam to escalate the pulpit and proclaim in the name of Allah, the All Merciful and Compassionate, there is no God but God and Muhammad is his Prophet.

The Sultan then touches the ground with his turbaned head—in a silent prayer. St Sophia is now a mosque.

Sultan Mehmet leaves the mosque and crosses the square to the old Palace of the Emperors, in ruins, founded by Constantine The Great 11 and ½ centuries before. He slowly wanders the ancient halls, his fine velvet slippers brushing the dust from the fabulous pebbled floor mosaics.

Then he murmurs two verses of a Persian poet:

As the spider weaves the curtain over the palace of the Roman Caesars

The owl sings the time of the house of Afrasiab

The Byzantine empire, founded by Constantine The Great on Monday, May 11, 330, was over on a Tuesday, May 29, 1453.

Sultan Mehmet is now the Lord of Constantinople and the Lord of the Ottoman Empire. He's only 21 years old.

BACK TO THE MAGIC MOUNTAIN

Last week, Turkish President Recep Tayyip Erdogan rechristened Hagia Sophia from a museum back into a mosque. He may have done it because his popularity is waning; his proxy wars are a disaster; his *Adalet ve Kalkınma Partisi* (AKP) party is shattered; and the economy is bleeding badly.

But what's striking is that right at the beginning of his official televised speech, Erdogan quoted exactly the same verses by the Persian poet murmured by Sultan Mehmet in that fateful afternoon in 1453.

Erdogan's latest move—which is part of his perennial master

plan to claim leadership of global Islam over the decrepit House of Saud—was widely interpreted in myriad latitudes as yet another instance of clash of civilizations: not only Orthodox Christianity vs. Islam but once again East vs. West.

That reminded me of another East vs. West recent derivation: a revival of the Settembrini vs. Naphta debate in Thomas Mann's *The Magic Mountain*, promoted by a Dutch think tank, the Nexus Institute, which aims to "keep the spirit of European humanism alive". The debate pitted Aleksander Dugin against Bernard-Henri Levy (widely known in France as BHL). The full transcript of the debate is here.[120]

Dugin is a leading Eurasianist and the conceptualizer of the— largely banned in the West—Fourth Political Theory. [121] As a philosopher and political theorist, Dugin is cartoonishly demonized across the West as "Putin's brain", a closet fascist and "the most dangerous philosopher in the world".

BHL, hailed as "one of the West's leading intellectuals", is a vain poseur who emerged as a "*nouveau philosophe*" in the mid-1970s and ritually regurgitates the usual Atlanticist mantras enveloped in flowery quotes. He managed, among other feats, to write a book about Pakistan without knowing anything whatsoever about Pakistan, as I thrashed it on *Asia Times* back in 2002.

Here are a few interesting talking points throughout the debate.

Dugin stresses the end of Western hegemony and global liberalism. He asks BHL, directly, how, "interestingly, in your book, you define the American empire or the global liberal system as a system of nihilism, based on nothing."[122] Dugin does define himself as a nihilist "in the sense that I refuse the universality of

---

[120] https://www.geopolitica.ru/en/article/return-settembrini-and-naphta-21st-century

[121] https://arktos.com/product/the-fourth-political-theory

[122] https://www.amazon.com/Empire-Five-Kings-Americas-Abdication-ebook/dp/B07F6914X3/ref=sr_1_1?keywords=The+Five+Kings+Bernard-Henri+Levi&qid=1594876741&sr=8-1

modern Western values (...) I just challenge that the only way to interpret democracy is as the rule of minorities against the majority, that the only way to interpret freedom is as individual freedom, and that the only way to interpret human rights is by projecting a modern, Western, individualistic version of what it means to be human on other cultures."

BHL, which seems not to have read his own, dreary, book—this is something Dugin told me in person last year in Beirut, after the debate—prefers to resort to proverbial, infantile Putin bashing, picked up over and over again, stressing "there is a bad, dark wind of nihilism in its proper sense, which is a Nazi and a fascist sense, which is blowing in the great Russia."

Later on in the debate, BHL adds, "I really believe that there is a link between, on the one side, your and Huntington's way of thinking; and, on the other side, the occupation of Crimea, the 30,000 deaths in Ukraine and the war in Syria with its bloodbath, tragic and horrible."

On racism, Dugin is adamant: he does not defend it. For him, "Racism is an Anglo-Saxon liberal construction based on a hierarchy between peoples. I think this is criminal." Then he defines "a new Manichean division, a new racism. Those who are in favor of Western values, they are good. Everybody who challenges that, in the Islamic tradition, in the Russian tradition, in the Chinese tradition, in the Indian tradition, everywhere, they are populists, and they are classified as fascism. I think that is a new kind of racism."

BHL prefers to concentrate on "the civilization of human rights, freedom, individual dignity, and so on. This deserves to be universalized. This should be conceived, except if you are a racist, as profitable for the entire humanity." And then it's anti-Semitism all over again: "All the men who you quoted and from whom you draw your inspiration—Spengler, Heidegger, who is also a great philosopher of course, and others—are contaminated, corrupted, infected by this plague which is antisemitism. And alas—you too."

In Paris circles, the joke is that the only thing BHL cares about is the promotion of BHL. And everyone who does not agree with one of the "leading Western intellectuals" is Anti-Semitic.

BHL insists he's interested in building bridges. But it's Dugin who frames the real heart of the matter: "When we try to build bridges too early, without knowing the structure of the Other—the problem is the Other. The West doesn't understand the Other as something positive. It is all the same, and we immediately try to find bridges—they are illusions, and not bridges, because we are projecting ourselves. The Other is the same, the ideology of the same. We first need to understand otherness."

BHL totally ignores Levi-Strauss. It's Dugin who refers to Levi-Strauss when talking about The Other, describing him as one of his teachers:

"This anthropological pluralism, I agree, is precisely the American and French tradition. But it is not reflected in politics, or it is reflected in a very perverted way. So I think there is a big contradiction between this anthropological thought in American universities and French universities, and a kind of very aggressive colonial neo-imperialist form to promote American interests on the world scale with weapons."

BHL is left with—what else—Putin demonization: "The real imperialism, the real one who is interfering and sowing disorder and interfering in the affairs of others, alas, is Putin. And I need not speak of America, where it is now proved that there has been a huge, crude, and evident Russian intervention in the electoral process of the last election." BHL, who does not even qualify as a neophyte in geopolitics, is oblivious to the absolute debunking of Russiagate.

BHL is adamant "there is today a real clash of civilizations. But not the one you mention in your books, between the north and the east and the west and the south and all of that; there is a clash of civilizations all over the planet between those who believe in human rights, in liberty, in the right for a body not to be tortured and martyred, and those who are happy with illiberalism and the revival of authoritarianism and slavery."

Dugin's challenge for years has been to try to conceptualize what may come next, after the failure of Marxism, fascism and liberal democracy. As much as he thinks Eurasian, he's inclusive—incorporating "Euro" with "Asia". BHL for his part simplistically reduces every "evil" to "illiberalism", where Russia, China, Iran and Turkey—no nuances—are thrown in the same dustbin alongside the vacuous and actually murderous House of Saud.

MAO RETURNS

Now let's attempt a light-hearted ending to our mini-triptych on the clash of civilizations. Inevitably, that has to do with the ongoing US-China Hybrid War.

Around two years ago, the following dialogue was a smash hit on Chinese Weibo. The Great Helmsman Mao Zedong—or his ghost—was back in town, and he wanted to know about everything that was goin' on. Call it a—revisionist?—realpolitik version of the clash of civilizations.

Mao. Can the people eat their fill?

Answer. There's so much to eat they're dieting.

Mao. Are there still any capitalists?

Answer. They're all doing business overseas now!

Mao. Do we produce more steel than England?

Answer. Tangshan alone produces more than America.

Mao. Did we beat social imperialism (as in the former USSR)?

Answer. They dissolved it themselves!

Mao. Did we smash imperialism?

Answer. We're the imperialists now!

Mao. And what about my Cultural Revolution?

Answer. It's in America now!"

Asia Times, July 2020

20. SHADOWPLAY REVISITED: HOW EURASIA IS BEING RESHAPED

We have seen how China is meticulously planning all its crucial geopolitical and geoeconomic moves all the way to 2030 and beyond.

What you are about to read next comes from a series of private, multilateral discussions among intel analysts, and may helpfully design the contours of the Big Picture.

In China, it's clear the path ahead points to boosting internal demand, and shifting monetary policy towards the creation of credit to consolidate the building of world-class domestic industries.

In parallel, there's a serious debate in Moscow that Russia should proceed along the same path. As an analyst puts it, "Russia should not import anything but technologies it needs until it can create them themselves and export only the oil and gas that is required to pay for imports that should be severely restricted. China still needs natural resources, which makes Russia and China unique allies. A nation should be as self-sufficient as possible."

That happens to mirror the exact Chinese Communist Party (CCP) strategy, as delineated by President Xi in his July 31 Central Committee meeting. [123]

And that also goes right against a hefty neoliberal wing in the CCP—collaborationists?—who would dream of a party conversion into Western-style social democracy, on top of it subservient to the interests of Western capital.

Comparing China's economic velocity now with the US is like comparing a Maserati Gran Turismo Sport (with a V8 Ferrari engine) with a Toyota Camry. China, proportionately, holds a larger reservoir of very well educated young generations; an

---

[123] https://asiatimes.com/2020/08/everything-going-according-to-plan-in-china/

accelerated rural-urban migration; increased poverty eradication; more savings; a cultural sense of deferred gratification; more—Confucianist—social discipline; and infinitely more respect for the rationally educated mind. The process of China increasingly trading with itself will be more than enough to keep the necessary sustainable development momentum going.

THE HYPERSONIC FACTOR

Meanwhile, on the geopolitical front, the consensus in Moscow—from the Kremlin to the Foreign Ministry—is that the Trump administration is not "agreement-capable", a diplomatic euphemism that refers to a de facto bunch of liars; and it's also not "legal-capable", an euphemism applied, for instance, to lobbying for snapback sanctions when Trump has already ditched the JCPOA.

President Putin has already said in the recent past that negotiating with Team Trump is like playing chess with a pigeon: the demented bird walks all over the chessboard, shits indiscriminately, knocks over pieces, declares victory, then runs away.

In contrast, serious lobbying at the highest levels of the Russian government is invested in consolidating the definitive Eurasian alliance, uniting Germany, Russia and China.

But that would only apply to Germany after Merkel. According to a US analyst, "the only thing holding back Germany is that they can expect to lose their car exports to the US and more, but I tell them that can happen right away because of the dollar-euro exchange rate, with the euro becoming more expensive."

On the nuclear front, and reaching way beyond the current Belarus drama—as in there will be no Maidan in Minsk—Moscow has made it very clear, in no uncertain terms, that any missile attack from NATO will be interpreted as a nuclear attack.

The Russian defensive missile system—including the already tested S-500s, and soon the already designed S-600s—arguably may be 99% effective. That means Russia would still have to absorb some punishment. And this is why Russia has built an extensive network of nuclear bomb shelters in big cities to protect at least 40 million people.

Russian analysts interpret China's defensive approach along the same lines. Beijing will want to develop—if they have not already done so—a defensive shield, and still retain the ability to strike back against a US attack with nuclear missiles.

The best Russian analysts, such as Andrei Martyanov, know that the three top weapons of a putative next war will be offensive and defensive missiles and submarines combined with cyber warfare capabilities.

The key weapon today—and the Chinese understand it very clearly—is nuclear submarines. Russians are observing how China is building their submarine fleet—carrying hypersonic missiles—faster than the US. Surface fleets are obsolete. A wolf pack of Chinese submarines can easily knock out a carrier task force. Those 11 US carrier task forces are in fact worthless.

So in the—horrifying—event of the seas becoming un-sailable in a war, with the US, Russia and China blocking all commercial traffic, that's the key strategic reason pushing China to obtain as much of its natural resources overland from Russia.

Even if pipelines are bombed they can be fixed in no time. Thus the supreme importance for China of Power of Siberia—as well as the dizzying array of Gazprom projects. [124]

THE HORMUZ FACTOR

A closely guarded secret in Moscow is that right after German sanctions imposed in relation to Ukraine, a major global energy operator approached Russia with an offer to divert to China no less than 7 million barrels a day of oil plus natural gas. Whatever happens, the stunning proposal is still sitting on the table of Shmal Gannadiy, a top oil/gas adviser to President Putin.

In the event that would ever happen, it would secure for China all the natural resources they need from Russia. Under this hypothesis, the Russian rationale would be to bypass German sanctions by switching its oil exports to China, which from a Russian point of view is more advanced in consumer technology

---

[124] https://www.gazprom.com/projects/

than Germany.

Of course this all changed with the imminent conclusion of Nord Stream 2—despite Team Trump taking no prisoners to sanction everyone in sight.

Backdoor intel discussions made it very clear to German industrialists that if Germany would ever lose its Russian source of oil and natural gas, coupled with the Strait of Hormuz shut down by Iran in the event of an American attack, the German economy might simply collapse.

There have been serious cross-country intel discussions about the possibility of a US-sponsored October Surprise involving a false flag to be blamed on Iran. Team Trump's "maximum pressure" on Iran has absolutely nothing to do with the JCPOA. What matters is that even indirectly, the Russia-China strategic partnership has made it very clear that Tehran will be protected as a strategic asset—and as a key node of Eurasia integration.

Cross-intel considerations center on a scenario assuming a—quite unlikely—collapse of the government in Tehran. The first thing Washington would do in this case is to pull the switch of the Society for Worldwide Interbank Financial Telecommunication (SWIFT) clearing system. The target would be to crush the Russian economy. That's why Russia and China are actively increasing the merger of the Russian Mir and the Chinese CIPS payment systems, as well as bypassing the US dollar in bilateral trade.

It has already been gamed in Beijing that were that scenario ever to take place, China might lose its two key allies in one move, and then have to face Washington alone, still on a stage of not being able to assure for itself all the necessary natural resources. That would be a real existential threat. And that explains the rationale behind the increasing interconnection of the Russia-China strategic partnership plus the $400 billion, 25-year-long China-Iran deal.

BISMARCK IS BACK

Another possible secret deal already discussed at the highest intel levels is the possibility of a Bismarckian Reinsurance Treaty to be established between Germany and Russia. The inevitable consequence would be a de facto Berlin-Moscow-Beijing alliance spanning the Belt and Road Initiative, alongside the creation of a new—digital?—Eurasian currency for the whole Eurasian alliance, including important yet peripheral actors such as France and Italy.

Well, Beijing-Moscow is already on. Berlin-Beijing is a work in progress. The missing link is Berlin-Moscow.

That would represent not only the ultimate nightmare for Mackinder-drenched Anglo-American elites, but in fact the definitive passing of the geopolitical torch from maritime empires back to the Eurasian heartland.

It's not a fiction anymore. It's on the table.

Adding to it, let's do some little time traveling and go back to the year 1348.

The Mongols of the Golden Horde are in Crimea, laying siege to Kaffa—a trading port in the Black Sea controlled by the Genoese.

Suddenly, the Mongol army is consumed by bubonic plague.

They start catapulting contaminated corpses over the walls of the Crimean city.

So imagine what happened when ships started sailing again from Kaffa to Genoa.

They transported the plague to Italy.

By 1360, the Black Death was literally all over the place—from Lisbon to Novgorod, from Sicily to Norway. As much as 60% of Europe's population may have been killed—over 100 million people.

A case can be made that the Renaissance, because of the plague, was delayed by a whole century.

COVID-19 is of course far from a medieval plague. But it's fair to ask.

What Renaissance could it be possibly delaying?

Well, it might well be actually advancing the Renaissance of Eurasia. It's happening just as the Hegemon, the former "end of history", is internally imploding, "distracted from distraction by distraction", to quote T.S. Eliot. Behind the fog, in prime shadowplay pastures, the vital moves to reorganize the Eurasian land mass are already on.

Asia Times, August 2020

21. From 9/11 to The Great Reset

9/11 was the foundation stone of the new millennium—ever as much indecipherable as the Mysteries of Eleusis. A year ago, on Asia Times, once again I raised a number of questions that still find no answer.

A lightning speed breakdown of the slings and arrows of outrageous (mis)fortune trespassing these two decades will certainly include the following:
The end of history. The short unipolar moment. The Pentagon's Long War. Homeland Security. The Patriot Act. Shock and Awe. The tragedy/debacle in Iraq. The 2008 financial crisis. The Arab Spring. Color revolutions. "Leading from behind". Humanitarian imperialism. Syria as the ultimate proxy war. The ISIS/Daesh farce. The JCPOA. Maidan. The Age of Psyops. The Age of the Algorithm. The Age of the 0.0001%.

Once again, we're deep in Yeats territory: "the best lack all conviction/ while the worst are full of passionate intensity."

All along, the "War on Terror"—the actual decantation of the Long War—proceeded unabated, killing Muslim multitudes and displacing at least 37 million people. [125]

WWII-derived geopolitics is over. Cold War 2.0 is in effect. It started as US against Russia, morphed into US against China and now, fully spelled out in the US National Security Strategy, and with bipartisan support, it's the US against both. The ultimate Mackinder-Brzezinski nightmare is at hand: the much dread "peer competitor" in Eurasia slouched towards the Beltway to be born in the form of the Russia-China strategic partnership.

Something's gotta give. And then, out of the blue, it did.

A drive by design towards ironclad concentration of power and

---

[125] https://watson.brown.edu/costsofwar/files/cow/imce/papers/2020-/Displacement_Vine%20et%20al_Costs%20of%20War%202020%2009%2008.pdf

geoconomic diktats was first conceptualized—under the deceptive cover of "sustainable development"—already in 2015 at the UN (here it is, in detail). [126]

Now, this new operating system—or technocratic digital dystopia—is finally being codified, packaged and "sold" since mid-summer via a lavish, concerted propaganda campaign.

WATCH YOUR MINDSPACE

The whole Planet Lockdown hysteria that elevated COVID-19 to postmodern Black Plague proportions has been consistently debunked, for instance here and here, drawing from the highly respected, original Cambridge source. [127], [128], [129]

The de facto controlled demolition of large swathes of the global economy allowed corporate and vulture capitalism, worldwide, to rake untold profits out of the destruction of collapsed businesses.

And all that proceeded with widespread public acceptance—an astonishing process of voluntary servitude.

None of it is accidental. As an example, over ten years ago, even before setting up a—privatized—Behavioral Insights Team, the British government was very much interested in "influencing" behavior, in collaboration with the London School of Economics and Imperial College.

The end result was the MINDSPACE report.[130] That was all about behavioral science influencing policymaking and most of all, imposing neo-Orwellian population control.

126

/https://sustainabledevelopment.un.org/content/documents/21252030%20Agenda%20for%20Sustainable%20Development%20web.pdf

[127] https://www.rt.com/op-ed/500000-covid19-math-mistake-panic

[128] https://drmalcolmkendrick.org/2020/09/04/covid-why-terminology-really-matters/

[129] https://www.cambridge.org/core/journals/disaster-medicine-and-public-health-preparedness/article/public-health-lessons-learned-from-biases-in-coronavirus-mortality-overestimation/7ACD87D8FD2237285EB667BB28DCC6E9"

[130] https://www.bi.team/publications/mindspace/

MINDSPACE, crucially, featured close collaboration between Imperial College and the Santa Monica-based RAND corporation. Translation:

the authors of the absurdly flawed computer models that fed the Planet Lockdown paranoia working in conjunction with the top Pentagon-linked think tank.

In MINDSPACE, we find that, "behavioral approaches embody a line of thinking that moves from the idea of an autonomous individual, making rational decisions, to a 'situated' decision-maker, much of whose behavior is automatic and influenced by their 'choice environment'".

So the key question is who decides what is the "choice environment." As it stands, our whole environment is now conditioned by COVID-19. Let's call it "the disease". And that is more than enough to beautifully set up "the cure": The Great Reset. [131]

THE BEATING HEART

The Great Reset was officially launched in early June by the World Economic Forum—the natural habitat of Davos Man. Its conceptual base is something the WEF describes as Strategic Intelligence Platform: "a dynamic system of contextual intelligence that enables users to trace relationships and interdependencies between issues, supporting more informed decision-making".

It's this platform that promotes the complex crossover and interpenetration of COVID-19 and the Fourth Industrial Revolution—conceptualized back in December 2015 and the WEF's choice futuristic scenario.[132] One cannot exist without the other. That is meant to imprint in the collective unconscious—at least in the West—that only the WEF-sanctioned "stakeholder" approach is capable of solving the COVID-19 challenge.

The Great Reset is immensely ambitious, spanning over 50

---

[131] https://www.weforum.org/focus/the-great-reset
[132] https://www.foreignaffairs.com/articles/2015-12-12/fourth-industrial-revolution

fields of knowledge and practice.[133] It interconnects everything from economy recovery recommendations to "sustainable business models", from restoration of the environment to the redesign of social contracts.

The beating heart of this matrix is—what else—the Strategic Intelligence Platform, encompassing, literally, everything: "sustainable development", "global governance", capital markets, climate change, biodiversity, human rights, gender parity, LGBTI, systemic racism, international trade and investment, the— wobbly—future of the travel and tourism industries, food, air pollution, digital identity, blockchain, 5G, robotics, artificial intelligence.

In the end, only an all-in-one Plan A applies for making these systems interact seamlessly: the Great Reset—shorthand for a New World Order that has always been glowingly evoked, but never implemented. There is no Plan B.

THE COVID-19 "LEGACY"

The two main actors behind the Great Reset are Klaus Schwab, the WEF's founder and executive chairman, and International Monetary Fund (IMF) Managing Director Kristalina Georgieva. Georgieva is adamant that "the digital economy is the big winner of this crisis". She believes the Great Reset must imperatively start in 2021.

The House of Windsor and the UN are prime executive co-producers. Top sponsors include BP, Mastercard and Microsoft. It goes without saying that everyone who knows how complex geopolitical and geoeconomic decisions are taken is aware that these two main actors are just reciting a script. Call the authors "the globalist elite". Or, in praise of Tom Wolfe, the Masters of the Universe.

Schwab, predictably, wrote the Great Reset's mini-manifesto. [134]Over a month later, he expanded on the absolutely key

---

[133] https://www.weforum.org/agenda/2020/04/strategic-intelligence-widget-artificial-intelligence-audience-content/

[134] https://www.weforum.org/agenda/2020/06/now-is-the-time-for-a-

connection: the "legacy" of COVID-19.[135]

All this has been fully fleshed in a book, co-written with Thierry Malleret, who directs the WEF's Global Risk Network.[136] COVID-19 is described as having "created a great disruptive reset of our global, social, economic and political systems". Schwab spins COVID-19 not only as a fabulous "opportunity", but actually as the *creator* of the—now inevitable—Reset.

All that happens to dovetail beautifully with Schwab's own baby: COVID-19 "accelerated our transition into the age of the Fourth Industrial Revolution". The revolution has been extensively discussed at Davos since 2016.

The book's central thesis is that our most pressing challenges concern the environment—considered only in terms of climate change—and technological developments, which will allow the expansion of the Fourth Industrial Revolution.

In a nutshell, the WEF is stating that corporate globalization, the hegemonic modus operandi since the 1990s, is dead. Now it's time for "sustainable development"—with "sustainable" defined by a select group of "stakeholders", ideally integrated into a "community of common interest, purpose and action."

Sharp Global South observers will not fail to compare the WEF's rhetoric of "community of common interest" with the Chinese "community of shared interests" as applied to the Belt and Road Initiative, which is a de facto continental trade/development project.

The Great Reset presupposes that all stakeholders—as in the whole planet—must toe the line. Otherwise, as Schwab stresses, we will have "more polarization, nationalism, racism, increased social unrest and conflicts".

So this is—once again—a "you're with us or against us" ultimatum, eerily reminiscent of our old 9/11 world. Either the Great Reset is peacefully established, with whole nations dutifully obeying the new guidelines designed by a bunch of self-appointed

---

great-reset/
[135] https://www.weforum.org/agenda/2020/07/covid19-this-is-how-to-get-the-great-reset-right/
[136] https://www.amazon.com/dp/2940631123

neo-Platonic Republic sages, or it's chaos.

Whether COVID-19's ultimate "window of opportunity" presented itself as a mere coincidence or by design, will always remain a very juicy question.

DIGITAL NEO-FEUDALISM

The actual, face-to-face Davos meeting next year has been postponed to the summer of 2021. But virtual Davos will proceed in January, focused on the Great Reset.

Already three months ago, Schwab's book hinted that the more everyone is mired in the global paralysis, the more it's clear that things will never be *allowed* to return to what we considered normal.

Five years ago, the UN's Agenda 2030—the Godfather of the Great Reset—was already insisting on vaccines for all, under the patronage of the WHO and CEPI—co-founded in 2016 by India, Norway and the Bill and Belinda Gates foundation.[137]

Timing could not be more convenient for the notorious Event 201 "pandemic exercise" in October last year in New York, with the Johns Hopkins Center for Health Security partnering with—who else—the WEF and the Bill and Melinda Gates Foundation.[138] No in-depth criticism of Gates's motives is allowed by media gatekeepers because, after all, he finances them.[139]

What has been imposed as an ironclad consensus is that without a COVID-19 vaccine there's no possibility of anything resembling normality.

And yet a recent, astonishing paper published in Virology Journal—which also publishes Dr. Fauci's musings—unmistakably demonstrates that "chloroquine is a potent inhibitor of SARS coronavirus infection and spread".[140] This is a "relatively

---

[137] https://cepi.net
[138] https://www.centerforhealthsecurity.org/event201/
[139] https://www.cjr.org/criticism/gates-foundation-journalism-funding.php
[140] https://virologyj.biomedcentral.com/articles/10.1186/1743-422X-2-69

safe, effective and cheap drug" whose "significant inhibitory antiviral effect when the susceptible cells were treated either prior to or after infection suggests a possible prophylactic and therapeutic use."

Even Schwab's book admits that COVID-19 is "one of the least deadly pandemics in the last 2000 years" and its consequences "will be mild compared to previous pandemics".

It doesn't matter. What matters above all is the "window of opportunity" offered by COVID-19, boosting, among other issues, the expansion of what I previously described as Digital Neo-Feudalism—or Algorithm gobbling up Politics.[141] No wonder politico-economic institutions from the WTO to the EU as well as the Trilateral Commission are already investing in "rejuvenation" processes, code for even more concentration of power.

SURVEY THE IMPONDERABLES

Very few thinkers, such as German philosopher Hartmut Rosa, see our current plight as a rare opportunity to "decelerate" life under turbo-capitalism. [142]

As it stands, the point is not that we're facing an "attack of the civilization-state". The point is assertive civilization-states—such as China, Russia, Iran—not submitted to the Hegemon, are bent on charting a quite different course. [143]

The Great Reset, for all its universalist ambitions, remains an insular, Western-centric model benefitting the proverbial 1%. Ancient Greece did not see itself as "Western". The Great Reset is essentially an Enlightenment-derived project. [144]

Surveying the road ahead, it will certainly be crammed with imponderables. From the Fed wiring digital money directly into

---

[141] https://www.strategic-culture.org/news/2020/05/15/how-biosecurity-is-enabling-digital-neo-feudalism/"
[142] https://www.mediapart.fr/journal/culture-idees/250820/hartmut-rosa-nous-sommes-devant-une-occasion-rare-de-decelerer
[143] https://www.noemamag.com/the-attack-of-the-civilization-state/
[144] https://www.strategic-culture.org/news/2020/08/31/the-dissolution-of-liberal-universalism/

smartphone financial apps in the US to China advancing an Eurasia-wide trade/economic system side-by-side with the implementation of the digital yuan.[145]

The Global South will be paying a lot of attention to the sharp contrast between the proposed wholesale deconstruction of the industrial economic order and the BRI project—which focuses on a new financing system outside of Western monopoly and emphasizes agro-industrial growth and long-term sustainable development.

The Great Reset would point to losers, in terms of nations, aggregating all the ones that benefit from production and processing of energy and agriculture, from Russia, China and Canada to Brazil, Indonesia and large swathes of Africa.

As it stands, there's only one thing we do know: the establishment at the core of the Hegemon and the drooling orcs of Empire will only adopt a Great Reset if that helps to postpone a decline accelerated on a fateful morning 19 years ago.

Asia Times, September 2020

---

[145] https://www.zerohedge.com/markets/preview-feds-coming-direct-money-transfers-brainard-says-fed-collaborating-mit-hypothetical

22. The Russia-China Vote

Whatever the geopolitical and geoeconomic consequences of the spectacular US dystopia, the Russia-China strategic partnership, in their own slightly different registers, have already voted on their path forward.

Here is how I framed what is at the heart of the Chinese 2021-2025 five-year plan approved at the plenum in Beijing last week. [146]

Here is a standard Chinese think tank interpretation. [147]

And here is some especially pertinent context examining how rampant Sinophobia is impotent when faced with an extremely efficient made in China model of governance.[148] This study shows how China's complex history, culture and civilizational axioms simply cannot fit into the Western, Christian hegemonic worldview.

The not so hidden "secret" of China's 2021-2025 five-year plan—which the Global Times described as "economic self-reliance"—is to base the civilization-state's increasing geopolitical clout on technological breakthroughs. [149]

Crucially, China is on a "self-driven" path—depending on little to no foreign input. Even a clear—"pragmatic"—horizon has been set: 2035, halfway between now and 2049.[150] By this time China should be on a par or even surpassing the US in geopolitical, geoeconomic and techno power.

That is the rationale behind the Chinese leadership actively

---

[146] https://www.strategic-culture.org/news/2020/10/30/can-you-smell-what-the-chinese-are-cooking/

[147] https://news.cgtn.com/news/2020-11-02/Why-China-s-five-year-plans-work--V5Gn4iu5vW/index.html

[148] https://laodan.blogspot.com/2020/09/the-ebook-first-societal-blow-in-late.html

[149] https://www.globaltimes.cn/content/1205337.shtml

[150] https://www.globaltimes.cn/content/1205131.shtml

studying the convergence of quantum physics and information sciences—which is regarded as the backbone of the Made in China push towards the Fourth Industrial Revolution.

The five-year plan makes it quite clear that the two key vectors are AI and robotics—where Chinese research is already quite advanced. Innovations in these fields will yield a matrix of applications in every area from transportation to medicine, not to mention weaponry.

Huawei is essential in this ongoing process, as it's not a mere data behemoth, but a hardware provider, creating platforms and the physical infrastructure for a slew of companies to develop their own versions of smart cities, safe cities—or medicines.

Big Capital—from East and West—is very much in tune with where all of this is going, a process that also implicates the core hubs of the New Silk Roads. In tune with the 21st century "land of opportunity" script, Big Capital will increasingly move towards East Asia, China and these New Silk hubs.

This new geoeconomic matrix will mostly rely on spin-offs of the Made in China 2025 strategy. A clear choice will be presented for most of the planet: "win-win" or "zero-sum."

THE FAILURES OF NEOLIBERALISM

After observing the mighty clash, enhanced by COVID-19, between the neoliberal paradigm and "socialism with Chinese characteristics", the Global South is only beginning to draw the necessary conclusions.

No Western propaganda tsunami can favorably spin what is in effect a devastating, one-two, ideological collapse.

Neoliberalism's abject failure in dealing with COVID-19 is manifestly evident all across the West.

The US election dystopia is now sealing the abject failure of Western liberal "democracy": what kind of "choice" is offered by Trump-Biden?

This is happening just as the ultra-efficient, relentlessly demonized "Chinese Communist Party" rolls out the road map for the next five years. Washington cannot even plan what happens the day ahead.

Trump's original drive, suggested by Henry Kissinger before the January 2017 inauguration, was to play—what else—Divide and Rule, seducing Russia against China.

This was absolute anathema for the Deep State and its Dem minions. Thus the subsequent, relentless demonization of Trump—with Russiagate topping the charts. And then Trump unilaterally chose to sanction and demonize China anyway.

Assuming a Dem victory, the scenario will veer towards Russia demonization on steroids even as hysterical Hybrid War on China will persist on all fronts—Uighurs, Tibet, Hong Kong, South China Sea, Taiwan.

Now compare all of the above with the Russian road map.

That was clearly stated in crucial interventions by Foreign Minister Sergey Lavrov and President Putin at the recent Valdai Club discussions.[151], [152]

Putin has made a key assertion on the role of Capital, stressing the necessity of "abandoning the practice of unrestrained and unlimited consumption—overconsumption—in favor of judicious and reasonable sufficiency, when you do not live just for today but also think about tomorrow."

Putin once again stressed the importance of the role of the state: "The state is a necessary fixture, there is no way [...] could do without state support."

And, in concert with the endless Chinese experimentation, he added that in fact there are no economic rules set in stone: "No model is pure or rigid, neither the market economy nor the command economy today, but we simply have to determine the level of the state's involvement in the economy. What do we use as a baseline for this decision? Expediency. We need to avoid using any templates, and so far, we have successfully avoided that."

Pragmatic Putin defined how to regulate the role of the state as "a form of art".

And he offered as an example, "keeping inflation up by a bit will make it easier for Russian consumers and companies to pay

---

[151] https://asiatimes.com/2020/10/iron-curtain-still-separates-russia-and-the-eu/

[152] http://en.kremlin.ru/events/president/news/64261

back their loans. It is economically healthier than the deflationary policies of western societies."

As a direct consequence of Putin's pragmatic policies—which include wide-ranging social programs and vast national projects—the West ignores that Russia may well be on the way to overtake Germany as the fifth largest economy in the world.

The bottom line is that, combined, the Russia-China strategic partnership is offering, especially to the Global South, two radically different approaches to the standard Western neoliberal dogma. And that, for the whole US establishment, is anathema.

So whatever the result of the Trump-Biden "choice", the clash between the Hegemon and the Top Two Sovereigns is only bound to become more incandescent.

Asia Times, November 2020

23. FLYING DRAGON, CRASHING EAGLE

Four geoeconomic summits compressed in one week tell the story of where we stand in these supremely dystopian times.

The (virtual) signing of the Regional Comprehensive Economic Partnership (RCEP) in Vietnam was followed by the equally virtual BRICS meeting hosted by Moscow, the Asia-Pacific Economic Cooperation (APEC) meeting hosted by Malaysia, and the G20 this past weekend hosted by Saudi Arabia. [153], [154]

Cynics have not failed to note the spectacular theater of the absurd of having the Top 20—at least in theory—economies discussing what is arguably the turning point in the world-system video-linked to a beheading-friendly desert oil hacienda with a 7th century mentality.

The Riyadh declaration did its best to lift the somber planetary mood, vowing to deploy "all available policy tools" (no precise details) to contain COVID-19 and heroically "save" the global economy by "advancing" global pandemic preparedness, vaccine development and distribution—in tandem with debt relief—for the Global South.[155]

Not a peep about The Great Reset—the Brave New World scheme concocted by Herr Schwab of Davos and fully supported by the IMF, Big Tech, transnational Big Capital interests and the oh so benign Prince Charles.[156] Meanwhile, off the record, G20 sherpas moaned about the lack of real global governance and multiple attacks on multilateralism.

And not a peep as well about the real life vaccine war between the expensive Western candidates—Pfizer, Moderna,

---

[153] https://asiatimes.com/2020/11/rcep-set-to-supercharge-the-new-silk-roads/
[154] https://g20.org/en/Pages/home.aspx
[155] https://www.g20riyadhsummit.org/pressroom/g20-riyadh-summit-leaders-declaration/
[156] https://www.weforum.org/great-reset/

AstraZeneca—and the much cheaper Russia-China versions—Sputnik V and Sinovac.[157]

What seems to be the case is that any agenda—sinister or otherwise—fits the one-size-fits-all vow by the G20 to provide "opportunities of the 21st century for all by empowering people, safeguarding the planet, and shaping new frontiers."

THE HOUSE OF XI

At the G20, President Xi Jinping did not waste the chance—after RCEP, BRICS and APEC—to once again emphasize China's priorities: multilateralism, support for WTO reform, ample international cooperation on vaccine research and production.

But then, in tandem with reducing tariffs and facilitating the trade of crucial medical supplies, Xi proposed a global health QR code—a sound way to restore global travel and trade: "While containing the virus, we need to restore the secure and smooth operation of global industrial and supply chains."

Predictably, there were howls about neo-Orwellian intrusion, comparing the QR code with the exceptionally misunderstood Chinese credit system. Herr Schwab's Great Reset in fact proposes something similar, with even more neo-Orwellian overtones, disguised under an innocent "Covid Pass" app, or highly secure "health passport".

What Xi has proposed amounts to just a mutual recognition of health certificates, issued by different nations, based on nucleic acid tests. No gene altering vaccines coupled with nanochips. These QR codes, incorporated to health apps, are already used for domestic travel in China.

Chinese officials have made it very clear that Beijing has been working as the representative of the Global South inside the G20. That's multilateralism in action. And the multilateralist drive extends from RCEP—signed between 15 nations—to the brilliant Sun Tzu maneuver of China now accepting even the Comprehensive and Progressive Agreement for Trans-Pacific Partnership (CPTPP), the successor of the Obama-promoted and

---

[157] https://tass.com/russia/1226499

Trump-detonated Trans-Pacific Partnership (TPP).

This revival—a case of Make TPP Chinese Again—can be envisaged because Beijing not only has mastered how to contain COVID-19 but is also recovering in lightning speed. China will be the only major economy growing in 2020—de facto leading the world to a tentative post-Covid paradigm.

What the APEC meeting made crystal clear is that with East Asia graphically hitting the economic limelight, as seen with RCEP, much vaunted US "leadership" inevitably diminishes.

APEC promoted a so-called Putrajaya Vision 2040, condensing an "open, dynamic, resilient and peaceful" Asia-Pacific all the way to 2040.[158] That neatly ties in with the three accumulated five-year Chinese plans all the way to 2035, approved last month at the CCP plenum in Beijing.

The emphasis, once again, is on multilateralism and an open global economy.

Few are more capable to capture the moment than Professor Wang Yiwei at the Institute of International Affairs at Renmin University, who wrote the best Chinese book on the Belt and Road Initiative. Wang stresses how China is in a period of "strategic opportunity" and is now "the most powerful leader of globalization". China's emphasis on multilateralism will "activate the connectivity and vitality of a trade platform like RCEP".

STRANGER THAN FICTION

Now compare all of the above with Trump at the G20 tweeting about the election dystopia and privileging golfing instead of discussing COVID-19 containment.

And then there's
The Elements of the China Challenge, the new 74-page delusional epic concocted by the office of Secretary Mike "We Lie, We Cheat, We Steal" Pompeo.[159] Diplomatic howls comparing it with the notorious George Kennan "long telegram" that codified

---

[158] https://www.globaltimes.cn/content/1207532.shtml"

[159] https://beta.documentcloud.org/documents/20407448-elements_of_the_china_challenge-20201117

the containment of the USSR in the Cold War are nonsense. Chinese Foreign Ministry reaction was more to the point: this was concocted by some "living fossils of the Cold War" and is doomed to end up "being consigned to the dustbin of history". [160]

President Xi Jinping, at RCEP, BRICS, APEC and the G20, concisely laid out the Chinese case: multilateralism, international cooperation on multiple fields, an open global economy, due representation of Global South's interests.

As we wait for a set of imponderables all the way to January 20, 2021, perhaps an angular approach to what may lie ahead for the world economy is best offered by fiction.

Enter *Billions*, season 5, episode 2, dialogue written by Andrew Ross Sorkin.

AXE. You know they call us traders "gamblers." The world's economy is one big casino, fueled by a giant debt bubble and computer driven derivatives. And there's only one thing better than being a gambler at a casino.

WAGS. That's being the house.

AXE. That's right. There's a systemized machine out there, sucking capital from localities and injecting it into the global markets, where it can be used to speculate and manipulate. And if something goes wrong there are bailouts and bail-ins, federal aid and easing. Where the government doesn't hunt you down, but instead gives you a nice soft net to land in.

WAGS. That's your answer to the fireside chat: You want to become a bank.

AXE. I want to become a bank.

WAGS. In order to rob it?

AXE. In order that I don't have to.

Asia Times, November 2020

---

[160] https://www.globaltimes.cn/content/1207403.shtml

24. OUR TECHNO-FEUDAL WORLD

The political economy of the Digital Age remains virtually *terra incognita*. In *Techno-Feudalism*,[161] published three months ago in France (no English translation yet), Cedric Durand, an economist at the Sorbonne, provides a crucial, global public service as he sifts through the new Matrix that controls all our lives.

Durand places the Digital Age in the larger context of the historical evolution of capitalism to show how the Washington consensus ended up metastasized into the Silicon Valley consensus. In a delightful twist, he brands the new groove as the "Californian ideology".

We're far away from Jefferson Airplane and the Beach Boys; it's more like Schumpeter's "creative destruction" on steroids, complete with

IMF-style "structural reforms" emphasizing "flexibilization" of work and outright marketization/financialization of everyday life.

The Digital Age was crucially associated with right-wing ideology from the very start. The incubation was provided by the Progress and Freedom Foundation (PFF), active from 1993 to 2010 and conveniently funded, among others, by Microsoft, AT&T, Disney, Sony, Oracle, Google and Yahoo.[162]

In 1994, PFF held a ground-breaking conference in Atlanta that eventually led to a seminal Magna Carta: literally, *Cyberspace and the American Dream: a Magna Carta for the Knowledge Era*, published in 1996, during the first Clinton term.[163]

---

[161] https.//www.amazon.com/Technof%C3%A9odalisme-French-C%C3%A9dric-DURAND-ebook/dp/B08GS8XV47/ref=pd_ybh_a_2?_encoding=UTF8&psc=1&refRID=ZCPCTPFZXYQBGGRPBDH3

[162] http://www.pff.org

[163] https://www.goodreads.com/book/show/39342741-cyberspace-and-the-american-dream

Not by accident the magazine *Wired* was founded, just like PFF, in 1993, instantly becoming the house organ of the "Californian ideology".

Among the authors of the Magna Carta we find futurist Alvin "Future Shock" Toffler and Reagan's former scientific counselor George Keyworth.[164] Before anyone else, they were already conceptualizing how "cyberspace is a bioelectronic environment which is literally universal". Their Magna Carta was the privileged road map to explore the new frontier.

THOSE RANDIAN HEROES

Also not by accident the intellectual guru of the new frontier was Ayn Rand and her quite primitive dichotomy between "pioneers" and the mob. Rand declared that egotism is good, altruism is evil, and empathy is irrational.

When it comes to the new property rights of the new El Dorado, all power should be exercised by the Silicon Valley "pioneers", a Narcissus bunch in love with their mirror image as superior Randian heroes. In the name of innovation they should be allowed to destroy any established rules, in a Schumpeterian "creative destruction" rampage.

That has led to our current environment, where Google, Facebook, Uber and co. can overstep any legal framework, imposing their innovations like a *fait accompli*.

Durand goes to the heart of the matter when it comes to the true nature of "digital domination": US leadership was never achieved because of spontaneous market forces.

On the contrary. The history of Silicon Valley is absolutely dependent on state intervention—especially via the industrial-military complex and the aero-spatial complex. The Ames Research Center, one of NASA's top labs, is in Mountain View. Stanford was always awarded juicy military research contracts. During WWII, Hewlett Packard, for instance, was flourishing thanks to their electronics being used to manufacture radars. Throughout the 1960s, the US military bought the bulk of the still

---

[164] https://www.tofflerassociates.com/about/the-toffler-legacy/

infant semiconductor production.

The Rise of Data Capital, a 2016 MIT Technological Review report produced "in partnership" with Oracle, showed how digital networks open access to a new, virgin underground brimming with resources: "Those that arrive first and take control obtain the resources they're seeking"—in the form of data. [165]

So everything from video-surveillance images and electronic banking to DNA samples and supermarket tickets implies some form of territorial appropriation. Here we see in all its glory the extractivist logic inbuilt in the development of Big Data.

Durand gives us the example of Android to illustrate the extractivist logic in action. Google made Android free for all smartphones so it would acquire a strategic market position, beating the Apple ecosystem and thus becoming the default internet entry point for virtually the whole planet. That's how a de facto, immensely valuable, online real estate empire is built.

The key point is that whatever the original business—Google, Amazon, Uber—strategies of conquering cyberspace all point to the same target: take control of "spaces of observation and capture" of data.

ABOUT THE CHINESE CREDIT SYSTEM...

Durand offers a finely balanced analysis of the Chinese credit system—a public/private hybrid system launched in 2013 during the 3rd plenum of the 18th Congress of the CCP, under the motto "to value sincerity and punish insincerity".

For the State Council, the supreme government authority in China, what really mattered was to encourage behavior deemed responsible in the financial, economic and socio-political spheres, and sanction what is not. It's all about trust. Beijing defines it as "a method of perfecting the socialist market economy system that improves social governance".

The Chinese term—*shehui xinyong*—is totally lost in translation in the West. Way more complex than "social credit",

---

[165] https://www.technologyreview.com/2016/03/21/161487/the-rise-of-data-capital/

it's more about "trustworthiness", in the sense of integrity. Instead of the pedestrian Western accusations of being an Orwellian system, priorities include the fight against fraud and corruption at the national, regional and local levels, violations of environmental rules, disrespect of food security norms.

Cybernetic management of social life is being seriously discussed in China since the 1980s. In fact, since the 1940s, as we see in Mao's *Little Red Book*. It could be seen as inspired by the Maoist principle of "mass lines", as in "start with the masses to come back to the masses: to amass the ideas of the masses (which are dispersed, non-systematic), concentrate them (in general ideas and systematic), then come back to the masses to diffuse and explain them, make sure the masses assimilate them and translate them into action, and verify in the action of the masses the pertinence of these ideas".

Durand's analysis goes one step beyond Soshana Zuboff's in *The Age of Surveillance Capitalism* when he finally reaches the core of his thesis, showing how digital platforms become "fiefdoms": they live out of, and profit from, their vast "digital territory" peopled with data even as they lock in power over their services, which are deemed indispensable.

And just as in feudalism, fiefdoms dominate territory by attaching serfs. Masters made their living profiting from the social power derived from the exploitation of their domain, and that implied unlimited power over the serfs.

It all spells out total concentration. Silicon Valley stalwart Peter Thiel has always stressed the target of the digital entrepreneur is exactly to bypass competition. As quoted in *Crashed: How a Decade of Financial Crises Changed the World*, Thiel declared, "Capitalism and competition are antagonistic. Competition is for losers."

So now we are facing not a mere clash between Silicon Valley capitalism and finance capital, but actually a new mode of production: a turbo-capitalist survival as rentier capitalism, where Silicon giants take the place of estates, and also the State. That is the "techno-feudal" option, as defined by Durand.

BLAKE MEETS BURROUGHS

Durand's book is extremely relevant to show how the theoretical and political critique of the Digital Age is still rarified. There is no precise cartography of all those dodgy circuits of revenue extraction. No analysis of how do they profit from the financial casino—especially mega investment funds that facilitate hyper-concentration. Or how do they profit from the hardcore exploitation of workers in the gig economy.

The total concentration of the digital glebe is leading to a scenario, as Durand recalls, already dreamed up by Stuart Mill, where every land in a country belonged to a single master. Our generalized dependency on the digital masters seems to be "the cannibal future of liberalism in the age of algorithms".

Is there a possible way out? The temptation is to go radical—a Blake/Burroughs crossover. We have to expand our scope of comprehension—and stop confusing the map (as shown in the Magna Carta) with the territory (our perception).

William Blake, in his proto-psychedelic visions, was all about liberation and subordination—depicting an authoritarian deity imposing conformity via a sort of source code of mass influence. Looks like a proto-analysis of the Digital Age.

William Burroughs conceptualized Control—an array of manipulations including mass media (he would be horrified by social media). To break down Control, we must be able to hack into and disrupt its core programs. Burroughs showed how all forms of Control must be rejected—and defeated: "Authority figures are seen for what they are: dead empty masks manipulated by computers".

Here's our future: hackers or slaves.

Asia Times, December 2020

25. KIM NO-VAX DOES DARPA

I have been going through my Asia Times archives selecting reports and columns for a new e-book on the Forever Wars—Afghanistan and Iraq. But then, out of the blue, I found this palimpsest, originally published by Asia Times in February 2014. It happened to be a Back to the Future exercise—traveling in time to survey the scene in the mid-1980s across Silicon Valley, MIT's AI lab, the Defense Advanced Research Projects Agency (DARPA) and the National Security Agency (NSA), weaving an intersection of themes, and a fabulous cast of characters, which prefigure the Brave New Techno World we're now immersed in, especially concerning the role of artificial intelligence. So this might be read today as a sort of preamble, or a background companion piece, to No Escape from our Techno-Feudal World, published early this month. Incidentally, everything that takes place in this account was happening a long 18 years before the end of the Pentagon's LifeLog project, run by DARPA, and the simultaneous launch of Facebook.[166] Enjoy the time travel.

In the spring of 1986, *Back to the Future*, the Michael J Fox blockbuster featuring a time-traveling DeLorean car, was less than a year old. The Apple Macintosh, launched via a single, iconic ad directed by Ridley (*Blade Runner*) Scott, was less than two years old. Ronald Reagan, immortalized by Gore Vidal as "the acting president," was hailing the mujahideen in Afghanistan as "freedom fighters."

---

[166] https://en.wikipedia.org/wiki/DARPA_LifeLog

The world was mired in Cyber Cold War mode; the talk was all about electronic counter-measures, with American C3s (command, control, communications) programmed to destroy Soviet C3s, and both the US and the USSR under MAD (mutually assured destruction) nuclear policies being able to destroy the earth 100 times over. Edward Snowden was not yet a three-year-old.

It was in this context that I set out to do a special report for a now-defunct magazine about artificial intelligence, roving from the Computer Museum in Boston to Apple in Cupertino and Pixar in San Rafael, and then to the campuses of Stanford, Berkeley and MIT.

AI had been "inaugurated" in 1956 by Stanford's John McCarthy and Marvin Minsky, a future MIT professor who at the time had been a student at Harvard. The basic idea, according to Minsky, was that any intelligence trait could be described so precisely that a machine could be created to simulate it.

My trip inevitably involved meeting a fabulous cast of characters. At MIT's AI lab, there was Minsky and also an inveterate iconoclast, Joseph Weizenbaum, who had coined the term "artificial intelligentsia" and believed computers could never "think" just like a human being.

At Stanford, there was Edward Feigenbaum, absolutely paranoid about Japanese scientific progress; he believed that if the Japanese developed a fifth-generation computer, based on artificial intelligence, that could think, reason and speak even such a difficult language as Japanese "the US will be able to bill itself as the first great post-industrial agrarian society."

And at Berkeley, still under the flame of hippie utopian populism, I found Robert Wilensky—Brooklyn accent, Yale gloss, California overtones; and philosopher Hubert Dreyfus, a tireless enemy of AI who got his kicks delivering lectures such as "Conventional AI as a Paradigm of Degenerated Research."

MEET KIM NO-VAX

Soon I was deep into Minsky's "frames"—a basic concept to organize every subsequent AI program—and the Chomsky paradigm: the notion that language is at the root of knowledge, and that formal syntax is at the root of language. That was the Bible of cognitive science at MIT.

Minsky was a serious AI enthusiast. One of his favorite themes was that people were afflicted with "carbon chauvinism": "This is central to the AI phenomenon. Because it's possible that more sophisticated forms of intelligence are not incorporated in cellular form. If there are other forms of intelligent life, then we may speculate over other types of computer structure."

At the MIT cafeteria, Minsky delivered a futurist rap without in the least resembling Dr Emmett Brown in Back to the Future:

"I believe that in less than five centuries we will be producing machines very similar to us, representing our thoughts and point of view. If we can build a miniaturized human brain weighing, let's say, one gram, we can lodge it in a spaceship and make it travel at the speed of light. It would be very hard to build a spaceship to carry an astronaut and all his food for 10,000 years of travel ... "

With Professor Feigenbaum, in Stanford's philosophical garden, the only space available was for the coming yellow apocalypse. But then one day I crossed Berkeley's post-hippie Rubicon and opened the door of the fourth floor of Evans Hall, where I met none other than Kim No-VAX.

No, that was not the Hitchcock blonde and Vertigo icon; it was an altered hardware computer (No-VAX because it had moved beyond Digital Equipment Corporation's VAX line of supercomputers), financed by the mellifluously-acronymed Pentagon military agency DARPA, decorated with a photo of Kim Novak and humming with the sexy vibration of—at the time immense—2,900 megabytes of electronic data spread over its body.

The US government's DARPA was all about computer science. In the mid-1980s, DARPA was immersed in a very ambitious program linking microelectronics, computer architecture and AI way beyond a mere military program. That was comparable to the

Japanese fifth-generation computer program. At MIT, the overwhelming majority of scientists were huge DARPA cheerleaders, stressing how the agency was leading research. Yet Terry Winograd, a computer science professor at Stanford, warned that had DARPA been a civilian agency, "I believe we would have made much more progress".

It was up to Professor Dreyfus to provide the voice of reason amidst so much cyber-euphoria:

> *"Computers cannot think like human beings because there's no way to represent all retrospective knowledge of an average human life—that is, 'common sense'—in a form that a computer may apprehend."* Dreyfus's drift was that with the boom of computer science, philosophy was dead—and he was a philosopher: *"Heidegger said that philosophy ended because it reached its apex in technology. Philosophy in fact reached its limit with AI. They, the scientists, inherited our questions. What is the mind? Now they have to answer for it. Philosophy is over."*

Yet Dreyfus was still teaching. Likewise at MIT, Weizenbaum was condemning AI as a racket for "lunatics and psychopaths"— but still continued to work at the AI lab.

NSA'S WET WEB DREAM

In no time, helped by these brilliant minds, I figured out that the AI "secret" would be a military affair, and that meant the National Security Agency—already in the mid-1980s vaguely known as "no such agency," with double the CIA's annual budget to pay for snooping on the whole planet.

The mission back then was to penetrate and monitor the global electronic net—that was years before all the hype over the "information highway"—and at the same time reassure the Pentagon over the inviolability of its lines of communication. For those comrades—remember, the Cold War, even with Gorbachev in power in the USSR, was still on—AI was a gift from God (beating Pope Francis by almost three decades).

So what was the Pentagon/NSA up to, at the height of the Star Wars hype, and over a decade and a half before the Revolution in Military Affairs (RMA) and the Full Spectrum Dominance doctrine?

They already wanted to control their ships and planes and heavy weapons with their voices, not their hands; voice command a la Hal, the star computer in Stanley Kubrick's *2001: A Space Odyssey*. Still, that was a faraway dream. Minsky believed that "only in the next century" would we be able to talk to a computer. Others believed that would never happen. Anyway, IBM was already working on a system accepting dictation; and MIT on another system that identified words spoken by different people; while Intel was developing a special chip for all this.

Although, predictably, prevented from visiting the NSA, I soon learned that the Pentagon was expecting to possess "intelligent" computing systems by the 1990s; Hollywood, after all, already had unleashed the *Terminator* series. It was up to Professor Wilensky, in Berkeley, to sound the alarm bells:

"Human beings don't have the appropriate engineering for the society they developed. Over a million years of evolution, the instinct of getting together in small communities, belligerent and compact, turned out to be correct. But then, in the 20th century, man ceased to adapt. Technology overtook evolution. The brain of an ancestral creature, like a rat, which sees provocation in the face of every stranger, is the brain that now controls the earth's destiny."

It was as if Wilensky was describing the NSA as it would be 28 years later. Some questions still remain unanswered; for instance, if our race does not fit anymore the society it built, who'd guarantee that its machines are properly engineered? Who'd guarantee that intelligent machines act in our interest?"

What was already clear by then was that "intelligent" computers would not end a global arms race. And it would be a long time, up to the Snowden revelations in 2013, for most of the planet to have a clearer idea of how the NSA orchestrates the Orwellian-Panopticon complex. As for my back to the future trip, in the end I did not manage to uncover the "secret" of AI. But I'll always remain very fond of Kim No-VAX.

Asia Times, December 2020

26. Soleimani Geopolitics, One Year On

One year ago, the Raging Twenties started with a murder. [167] The assassination of Maj Gen Qassem Soleimani, commander of the Quds Force of the Islamic Revolutionary Guards Corps (IRGC), alongside Abu Mahdi al-Muhandis, the deputy commander of Iraq's Hashd al-Sha'abi militia, by laser-guided Hellfire missiles launched from two MQ-9 Reaper drones, was an act of war.

Not only the drone strike at Baghdad airport, directly ordered by President Trump, was unilateral, unprovoked and illegal: it was engineered as a stark provocation, to detonate an Iranian reaction that would then be countered by American "self-defense", packaged as "deterrence". Call it a perverse form of double down, reversed false flag.

The imperial Mighty Wurlitzer spun it as a "targeted killing", a pre-emptive op squashing Soleimani's alleged planning of "imminent attacks" against US diplomats and troops.

False. No evidence whatsoever. And then, Iraqi Prime Minister Adil Abdul-Mahdi, in front of his Parliament, offered the ultimate context: Soleimani was on a diplomatic mission, on a regular flight between Damascus and Baghdad, involved in complex negotiations between Tehran and Riyadh, with the Iraqi Prime Minister as mediator, at the request of President Trump.

So the imperial machine—in complete mockery of international law—assassinated a de facto diplomatic envoy.

The three top factions who pushed for Soleimani's assassination were US neocons—supremely ignorant of Southwest Asia's history, culture and politics—and the Israeli and Saudi lobbies, who ardently believe their interests are advanced every time Iran is attacked. Trump could not possibly see The Big

---

[167] https://asiatimes.com/2020/01/us-starts-the-raging-twenties-declaring-war-on-iran/

Picture and its dire ramifications: only what his major Israeli-firster donor Sheldon Adelson dictates, and what Jared of Arabia Kushner whispered in his ear, remote-controlled by his close pal Muhammad bin Salman (MbS).

THE ARMOR OF AMERICAN "PRESTIGE"

The measured Iranian response to Soleimani's assassination was carefully calibrated to not detonate vengeful imperial "deterrence": precision missile strikes on the American-controlled Ain al-Assad air base in Iraq. The Pentagon received advance warning.

Predictably, the run-up towards the first anniversary of Soleimani's assassination had to degenerate into intimations of US-Iran once again on the brink of war.

So it's enlightening to examine what the Commander of the IRGC Aerospace Division, Brigadier General Amir-Ali Hajizadeh, told [168] Lebanon's Al Manar network: "The US and the Zionist regime [Israel] have not brought security to any place and if something happens here (in the region) and a war breaks out, we will make no distinction between the US bases and the countries hosting them."

Hajizadeh, expanding on the precision missile strikes a year ago, added, "We were prepared for the Americans' response and all our missile power was fully on alert. If they had given a response, we would have hit all of their bases from Jordan to Iraq and the Persian Gulf and even their warships in the Indian Ocean."

The precision missile strikes on Ain al-Assad, a year ago, represented a middle-rank power, enfeebled by sanctions, and facing a huge economic/financial crisis, responding to an attack by targeting imperial assets that are part of the Empire of Bases. That was a global first—unheard of since the end of WWII. It was clearly interpreted across vast swathes of the Global South as fatally piercing the decades-old hegemonic armor of American" prestige".

---

[168] https://www.tasnimnews.com/fa/news/1399/10/13/2423366/

So Tehran was not exactly impressed by two nuclear-capable B-52s recently flying over the Persian Gulf; or the US Navy announcing the arrival of the nuclear-powered, missile loaded USS Georgia in the Persian Gulf last week.

These deployments were spun as a response to an evidence-free claim that Tehran was behind a 21-rocket attack against the sprawling American embassy in Baghdad's Green Zone.

The (unexploded) 107mm caliber rockets—by the way marked in English, not Farsi—can be easily bought in some underground Baghdad souk by virtually anybody, as I have seen for myself in Iraq since the mid-2000s.

That certainly does not qualify as a casus belli—or "self-defense" merging with "deterrence". The CENTCOM justification actually sounds like a Monty Python sketch: an attack "…almost certainly conducted by an Iranian-backed rogue militia group."[169] Note that "almost certainly" is code for "we have no idea who did it".

How to Fight the—Real—War on Terror

Iranian Foreign Minister Javad Zarif did take the trouble to warn Trump, via Twitter, he was being set up for a fake casus belli—and blowback would be inevitable. That's a case of Iranian diplomacy being perfectly aligned with the IRGC: after all, the whole post-Soleimani strategy comes straight from Ayatollah Khamenei.

And that leads to the IRGC's Hajizadeh once again establishing the Iranian red line in terms of the Islamic Republic's defense: "We will not negotiate about the missile power with anyone"—pre-empting any move to incorporate missile reduction into a possible Washington return to the JCPOA. Hajizadeh has also emphasized that Tehran has restricted the range of its missiles to 2,000 km.

My friend Elijah Magnier, arguably the top war correspondent across Southwest Asia in the past four decades, has neatly detailed

---

[169] https://www.centcom.mil/MEDIA/STATEMENTS/Statements-View/Article/2456662/us-central-command-statement-on-dec-20-2020-rocket-attack/

the importance of Soleimani. [170]

Everyone not only along the Axis of Resistance—Tehran, Baghdad, Damascus, Hezbollah—but across vast swathes of the Global South is firmly aware of how Soleimani led the fight against ISIS/Daesh in Iraq from 2014 to 2015, and how he was instrumental in retaking Tikrit in 2015.

Zeinab Soleimani, the impressive General's daughter, has profiled the man, and the sentiments he inspired[171]. And Hezbollah's secretary-general Sayed Nasrallah, in an extraordinary interview, stressed Soleimani's "great humility", even "with the common people, the simple people."

Nasrallah tells a story that is essential to place Soleimani's modus operandi in the real—not fictional—war on terror, and deserves to be quoted in full: [173]

> At that time, Hajj Qassem traveled from Baghdad airport to Damascus airport, from where he came (directly) to Beirut, in the southern suburbs. He arrived to me at midnight. I remember very well what he said to me: "At dawn you must have provided me with 120 (Hezbollah) operation commanders." I replied "But Hajj, it's midnight, how can I provide you with 120 commanders?" He told me that there was no other solution if we wanted to fight (effectively) against ISIS, to defend the Iraqi people, our holy places [5 of the 12 Imams of Twelver Shi'ism have their mausoleums in Iraq], our Hawzas [Islamic seminars], and everything that existed in Iraq. There was no choice. "I don't need fighters. I need operational commanders [to supervise the Iraqi Popular Mobilization Units,

---

[170] https://ejmagnier.com/2021/01/01/iran-one-year-on-what-did-the-assassination-of-qassem-soleimani-achieve/
[171] https://www.youtube.com/watch?v=7Pz3fZNlCEQ
[172] https://video.moqawama.org/details.php?cid=1&linkid=2099
[173] https://resistancenews.org/2021/01/03/nasrallah-about-qassem-soleimani-and-his-victory-against-isis-in-iraq/

PMU]." This is why in my speech [about Soleimani's assassination], I said that during the 22 years or so of our relationship with Hajj Qassem Soleimani, he never asked us for anything. He never asked us for anything, not even for Iran. Yes, he only asked us once, and that was for Iraq, when he asked us for these (120) operations commanders. So he stayed with me, and we started contacting our (Hezbollah) brothers one by one. We were able to bring in nearly 60 operational commanders, including some brothers who were on the front lines in Syria, and whom we sent to Damascus airport [to wait for Soleimani], and others who were in Lebanon, and that we woke up from their sleep and brought in [immediately] from their house as the Hajj said he wanted to take them with him on the plane that would bring him back to Damascus after the dawn prayer. And indeed, after praying the dawn prayer together, they flew to Damascus with him, and Hajj Qassem traveled from Damascus to Baghdad with 50 to 60 Lebanese Hezbollah commanders, with whom he went to the front lines in Iraq. He said he didn't need fighters, because thank God there were plenty of volunteers in Iraq. But he needed [battle-hardened] commanders to lead these fighters, train them, pass on experience and expertise to them, etc. And he didn't leave until he took my pledge that within two or three days I would have sent him the remaining 60 commanders.

ORIENTALISM, ALL OVER AGAIN

A former commander under Soleimani that I met in Iran in 2018 had promised me and my colleague Sebastiano Caputo that he would try to arrange an interview with the Maj Gen—who never spoke to foreign media. We had no reason to doubt our interlocutor—so until the last Baghdad minute we were in this selective waiting list.

As for Abu Mahdi al-Muhandis, killed side by side with Soleimani in the Baghdad drone strike, I was part of a small group who spent an afternoon with him in a safe house inside—not outside—Baghdad's Green Zone in November 2017. My full report is here. [174]

Prof. Mohammad Marandi of the University of Tehran, reflecting on the assassination, told me, "the most important thing is that the Western view on the situation is very Orientalist. They assume that Iran has no real structures and that everything is dependent on individuals. In the West an assassination doesn't destroy an administration, company, or organization. Ayatollah Khomeini passed away and they said the revolution was finished. But the constitutional process produced a new leader within hours. The rest is history."

This may go a long way to explain Soleimani geopolitics. He may have been a revolutionary superstar—many across the Global South see him as the Che Guevara of Southwest Asia—but he was most of all a quite articulated cog of a very articulated machine.

The adjunct President of the Iranian Parliament, Hossein Amirabdollahian, told Iranian network Shabake Khabar that Soleimani, two years before the assassination, had already envisaged an inevitable "normalization" between Israel and Persian Gulf monarchies.

At the same time he was also very much aware of the Arab League 2002 position—shared, among others, by Iraq, Syria and Lebanon: a "normalization" cannot even begin to be discussed without an independent—and viable—Palestinian state under 1967 borders with East Jerusalem as capital.

Now everyone knows this dream is dead, if not completely buried. What remains is the usual, dreary slog: the American assassination of Soleimani, the Israeli assassination of top Iranian scientist Mohsen Fakhrizadeh, the relentless, relatively low-intensity Israeli warfare against Iran fully supported by the Beltway, Washington's illegal occupation of parts of northeast

---

[174] https://www.rt.com/news/409667-iraq-renaissance-muhandis-escobar/

Syria to grab some oil, the perpetual drive for regime change in Damascus, the non-stop demonization of Hezbollah.

BEYOND THE HELLFIRE

Tehran has made it very clear that a return to at least a measure of mutual respect between US-Iran involves Washington rejoining the JCPOA with no preconditions, and the end of illegal, unilateral Trump administration sanctions. These parameters are non-negotiable.

Nasrallah, for his part, in a speech in Beirut on Sunday, stressed,

> "one of the main outcomes of the assassination of General Soleimani and al-Muhandis is the calls made for the expulsion of US forces from the region. Such calls had not been made prior to the assassination. The martyrdom of the resistance leaders set US troops on the track of leaving Iraq."

This may be wishful thinking, because the military-industrial-security complex will never willingly abandon a key hub of the Empire of Bases.

More important is the fact that the post-Soleimani environment transcends Soleimani.

The Axis of Resistance—Tehran-Baghdad-Damascus-Hezbollah—instead of collapsing, will keep getting reinforced.

Internally, and still under "maximum pressure" sanctions, Iran and Russia will be cooperating to produce COVID-19 vaccines, and the Pasteur Institute of Iran will co-produce a vaccine with a Cuban company.[175]

Iran is increasingly solidified as the key node of the New Silk Roads in Southwest Asia: the Iran-China strategic partnership is constantly revitalized by FMs Zarif and Wang Yi, and that includes Beijing turbo-charging its geoeconomic investment in

---

[175] https://www.tehrantimes.com/news/456441/Iran-Cuba-coproducing-COVID-19-vaccine

South Pars—the largest gas field on the planet. [176]

Iran, Russia and China will be involved in the reconstruction of Syria—which will also include, eventually, a New Silk Road branch: the Iran-Iraq-Syria-Eastern Mediterranean railway.

All that is an interlinked, ongoing process no Hellfires are able to burn.

Asia Times, January 2021

---

[176] https://www.presstv.com/Detail/2020/10/10/636075/Zarif-Wang-Yi-Iran-China-Tengchong-partnership"

ABOUT THE AUTHOR

Pepe Escobar is a journalist, independent geopolitical analyst and author. Born in Brazil, he started in the daily newspaper business in 1982 as a music, cinema, literature and cultural critic and became a foreign correspondent in 1985, first in London and then Milan, Los Angeles and Paris.

In 1994 he decided to move from the West to Asia, first to Singapore and then Bangkok and Hong Kong. He has been living between Europe and Asia ever since—with bases alternating between London/Paris and Bangkok/Hong Kong, as well as stints in Washington and New York.

He has covered virtually everything important that happened across Asia in the past 25 years, including the geopolitics and geoeconomics of Southeast Asia, China, Russia, and progressively, the arc from Afghanistan/Pakistan to Central Asia, Iran, Iraq, Turkey and the Persian Gulf.

Switching from the "Asian miracle" to the "war on terror", after 9/11 he covered the wars on Afghanistan and Iraq (before, during and after), energy wars and, in the Obama years, the American "pivot" to Asia. For the past few years, his focus is the Chinese-driven New Silk Roads, all aspects of Eurasia integration, and the geopolitical clash between the US and the Russia/China strategic partnership.

He has written columns and Op-Eds for dozens of online publications—including Al Jazeera, RT and Sputnik—and has been a frequent guest of TV and radio shows from North America to Asia. His articles/columns are regularly translated in several languages.

He is currently a columnist/geopolitical analyst for Asia Times (Hong Kong), Consortium News (Washington) and Strategic Culture (Moscow).[177], [178], [179]

In Brazil, he published an experimental novel, *Speedball* (1987)

---

[177] https://www.asiatimes.com/
[178] https://consortiumnews.com/
[179] https://www.strategic-culture.org

and a book on the Asian miracle, *21st: the Asian Century* (1997). In the US, he published *Globalistan* (2007); *Red Zone Blues* (2007); *Obama does Globalistan* (2009); *Empire of Chaos* (2014); and *2030* (2015), all by Nimble Books. His 20-year archives on Asia Times are being released as a series of e-books. He currently lives between Paris and Bangkok.

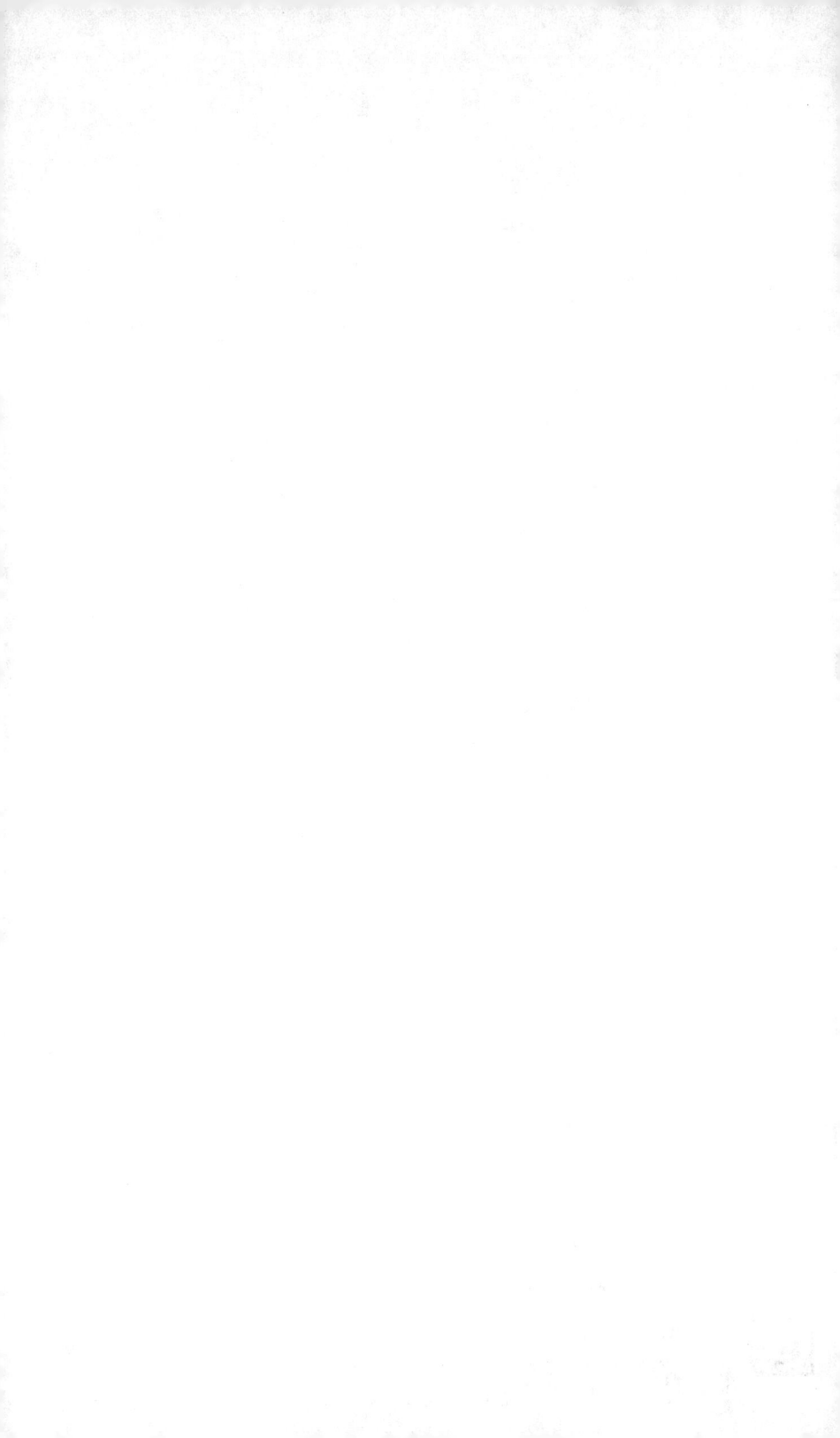

www.ingramcontent.com/pod-product-compliance
Lightning Source LLC
Chambersburg PA
CBHW071117160426
43196CB00013B/2594